Families on the Edge

Families on the Edge

Experiences of Homelessness and Care in Rural New England

Elizabeth Carpenter-Song

The MIT Press
Cambridge, Massachusetts
London, England

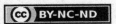
The MIT Press would like to thank the anonymous peer reviewers who provided comments on drafts of this book. The generous work of academic experts is essential for establishing the authority and quality of our publications. We acknowledge with gratitude the contributions of these otherwise uncredited readers.

This book was set in Stone Serif and Stone Sans by Westchester Publishing Services. Printed and bound in the United States of America.

Library of Congress Cataloging-in-Publication Data is available.

ISBN: 978-0-262-54618-8

10 9 8 7 6 5 4 3 2

Contents

Acknowledgments

The longitudinal research on which this book is based has been generously supported by numerous funders, including the Agency for Healthcare Research and Quality (AHRQ) (Career Development Award 1K12HS021695–01), the Claire Garber Goodman Fund for the Anthropological Study of Human Culture, the Columbia University Homelessness Prevention Scholars Program, the Dartmouth Synergy Community Engagement Pilot (NCATS 1UL1TR001086–04), and the Patient-Centered Outcomes Research Institute (PCORI) (Pipeline-to-Proposal Award 5108699).

I am deeply grateful to so many who contributed in different ways to this book. I thank Matthew Browne at the MIT Press and Neil Aggarwal, series editor for the Culture and Psychiatry Series at the MIT Press, for believing in this book project and supporting me through the process of writing and revision. I wish to thank the three anonymous reviewers who thoughtfully read and commented on the manuscript. I am grateful for your generous engagement, which has made the work undoubtedly stronger. I also thank the editors and peer reviewers of the journals in which previous versions of this research have been published. Portions of chapters 2 and 3 appeared in "Social Exclusion and Survival for Families Facing Homelessness in Rural New England," *Journal of Social Distress and the Homeless*, *25*(1) (2016), 41–52. Portions of chapter 5 appeared in "'The Kids Were My Drive': Shattered Families, Moral Striving, and the Loss of Parental Selves in the Wake of Homelessness," *Ethos*, *47*(1) (2019), 54–72. I have had the opportunity to present versions of this work at meetings of the American Anthropological Association, the Geisel School of Medicine Department of Psychiatry Grand Rounds, the Harvard Department of Global Health and Social Medicine Friday Morning Seminar, the Society for Psychological Anthropology, and the Upper Valley Haven. I thank my colleagues in these venues for your questions and comments, which have informed and deepened my thinking on lived experiences of housing insecurity, mental illness, and rural communities.

I am profoundly grateful to the five families that are the centerpiece of this work for allowing me into your lives and courageously sharing experiences of vulnerability with me. You have taught me so much about the struggles and joys of family life. I am humbled by your daily efforts to care for your families amid conditions of scarcity and suffering. I hope the words in these pages do your efforts justice and that this book can inform change for families that have experienced homelessness and mental health challenges. I thank the many other participants—those with lived experiences of homelessness, health and social service providers, legal advocates—who have contributed your perspectives and insights to inform this work.

I have benefitted from the wisdom of many mentors in the journey of this research. I thank Robert Welsch and Hoyt Alverson for first introducing me to medical anthropology and for the gift of your mentorship. Janis H. Jenkins, Mary-Jo DelVecchio Good, and Byron Good have deeply informed my approach to foregrounding lived experiences of suffering and engaging in the culture of medicine and psychiatry. I am beyond grateful to you all for believing in me and for always being there for me. Robert E. Drake welcomed me into the space of interdisciplinary mental health services research and has served as a model of what is possible in psychiatry by centering practice on the things that matter to people—work, family, and having a life. Sara Kobylenski, my community partner, served as a bridge to families and has been a deep collaborator in this work. By joining compassion with pragmatism, you have made a difference for so many families. I am so fortunate to have you all as guides in scholarship and in life.

Many dear colleagues and friends have discussed and read versions of this work over the years. Sienna Craig and Laura Ogden led ethnographic writing workshops in the department of anthropology at Dartmouth College that were enormously helpful in jumpstarting my writing at critical times and in offering a space of support and community. You have both been so helpful as I navigated new terrain in writing. I thank Anne Sosin, Renee Weeks, and Maryellen Griffin for reading this work and offering key perspectives from the spaces of public health, community-engaged research, trauma-informed care, and advocacy with marginalized populations. I thank

Manish K. Mishra for gifting me your insights from clinical practice and medical education and for the gift of your friendship. I'm grateful beyond words for our collaboration at the intersection of anthropology and medicine. I thank Ellen Kozelka for your careful read of my drafts and for sharing new scholarship in the anthropology of mental health and addiction. I thank Ken Sharpe for pushing my thinking regarding the role of systems and structures in the context of the issues presented in this book. I thank Michael Redmond for enabling continued collaborations.

I have had the delight of working with many students and recent graduates who supported this research in many ways—assisting with data collection and management, collaborating on participatory methods, and supporting manuscript preparation through literature searches and creating the figures that appear in this text. I thank Sadie Bronk, Jess Campanile, Charlotte Evans, Abbi Fischer, Allie Gerber, Connor Gibson, Ida Griesemer, Jay Kang, Taylor McKenna, John Torrey, Mia Winthrop, and Kaite Yang. I thank David Strickler, who worked as a research assistant on this project for many years, for his thoughtful engagement with the work of homelessness and mental health recovery in rural areas. I am grateful to the members of the Community Advisory Board for this project, Nicole Hopkins, Mark Marsh, and Lee Works. This group generously shared their perspectives and experiences to help translate the research findings into recommendations for practical action.

I wish to thank the many friends who have welcomed and nurtured my family in rural New England: Jessica and Ian Danner, Maegan and Sean Ellis, Larry and Patty Gould, Dawn and Todd Gunnerson, and John Risley and Alex Schroeder. Special thanks to Laura Doherty for reading every word. I'm profoundly grateful to you all for being my village. To my brothers, David Carpenter and Scott Carpenter, and their families thank you for your unending encouragement and support. I thank my parents, Alice Carpenter and James "Rick" Carpenter, for cultivating my curiosity, modeling a life of learning, and sacrificing to broaden the world of possibilities for me.

Finally, to my forever love, Arnold Song, and our amazing daughter, Maddy Song. You two are my world. Thank you for everything.

Prelude

Northern New England first took hold of me in the earliest days of my adulthood. As an 18-year-old, the rural Northeast beckoned me away from my suburban mid-Atlantic upbringing with its craggy granite mountains, winding two-lane roads, and small villages scattered across the landscape. Over the next five years, first as a student, then as a budding anthropologist, I took every opportunity to immerse myself in the place and its people. As a volunteer Big Sister, I came to know Northern New England through the experiences of one family, seeing up close the swirl of care, pressures of responsibility, tension, and joy in the tumbling flows of family life. I crossed more thresholds in rural and small-town New England as I followed visiting nurses into homes as they changed dressings on wounds and assisted people with the most intimate of care tasks, their hands strong and gentle as they lifted, bathed, and helped dress their patients. I knew, even then, that I was being given a special gift as strangers welcomed me to bear witness to their care.

I found myself gripped by this form of witnessing. While I had anticipated pursuing a clinical career, this expected trajectory was disrupted as I learned new ways of being with people during times of vulnerability and uncertainty. I followed my newfound path away from the hills and valleys of Northern New England to pursue my doctoral studies and postdoctoral training. In medical anthropology, I found the unique opportunity to bridge my longstanding interest in matters of health and illness with a discipline that requires contemplation, values aesthetics in its professional expression, and elevates our time with others as our windows into what it means to be human. As Byron Good (1994) has written:

> It is both the privilege and the obligation of medical anthropology to bring renewed attention to human experience, to suffering, to meaning and interpretation, to the role of narratives and historicity, as well as to the role of social formations and

institutions, as we explore a central aspect of what it means to be human across cultures. (p. 24)

Our methods of long-term immersion, involving relationships of deep trust, allow unique insights into what Arthur Kleinman has described as "what really matters" to people—that is, what is most at stake for particular people, at particular times, and in particular places (Kleinman, 1998, 2007). I have endeavored in the pages that follow in this book to illuminate—partially, imperfectly—what matters within and for families that have experienced multiple burdens of homelessness, mental illness, trauma, and substance use in Northern New England.

Writing about families, time folds in on itself as I remember my own childhood. As the youngest of three children, trailing my older brothers by nearly six and eight years, I always felt comfortable observing and listening. In grainy Super 8 footage, amid the wildly waving hands and mouths moving to express now silent words, I tend to be found at the edges of the frame. As I write this, it is nearly a year since I lost my mother, and I find myself awash in grief and gratitude. Long before my professors, my mother taught me how to be attuned to others and to pay attention to the details. Now, as I marvel at my own daughter, I share with her the lessons of learning to pause, to listen, and to be open to others.

I returned to Northern New England over a decade ago. Living in a small, rural town in New Hampshire, our family has learned the rhythms of the seasons: the bellwether of fall in a layer of fog across the fields and the first flame-tipped maple branches; winter air so cold the insides of your nose prickle with tiny icicles; the relief of spring quietly announced in snowdrops and daffodils bravely emerging from just-thawed ground; and summer—oh, summer—with the pink light of its long days yielding to cool nights and a soundtrack of cricket song. As transplants to New England, we have been supported by friends and neighbors always willing to lend a tool, give advice, or surprise us with bags heaping with fresh corn or a foil-wrapped package of cupcakes left on our porch. For our family, this has been a place of opportunity and belonging.

Yet I have also come to know other sides to rural New England through my work over the past decade. The families at the heart of this book have experienced harsh daily realities of struggling to survive in poverty, to take care of their families amid conditions of uncertainty and economic precarity, and to navigate through complex systems of care. They have entrusted me with their stories, which I share in the hope of sparking practical actions to make rural New England a place of opportunity for all families.

1 Introduction

As the sun filtered through the dense trees, my car's tires crunched along the winding gravel road leading up to Jim and Hannah's house. Fall had not yet closed in, and I soaked in September's warmth as everyone in New England does in the waning pages of summer before autumn's chapter brings a chill. The tinge of melancholy was deepened on this day because I knew that Jim and Hannah were facing another crisis that threatened to render them homeless again. A few months earlier, Jim had lost his job, sparking a cycle of falling behind on the rent payments for a small cabin tucked onto a Vermont hillside. This cabin was meant to be their fresh start, an opportunity to rebuild themselves in the wake of losing custody of their children and to sow a few seeds of stability on that patch of fertile land. Now months behind on their rent, they were seeing these promises quickly recede from view. Hannah was gripped by fear at the prospect of losing their home and had wept the last time I saw her as we sipped cans of Coca-Cola on the small front porch. "What are we going to do? I'm lost. Stuck. Numb. Like watching myself in a movie. You know it's reality, but it's like you're watching yourself."

Yet the despair that had marked our last meeting did not prepare me for the scene I was about to enter. As I turned my blue Toyota Corolla into the driveway, I noticed an unfamiliar car parked outside of the house. I got out of my car and walked up the gravel driveway, where I found Hannah sitting in her truck. Her eyes were wild when I greeted her: "My landlord's here." She got out of the truck, slamming the door. Hannah paced, watching as her landlord led a somber parade with his wife as they carried boxes and laundry baskets heaped with Hannah and Jim's belongings out of the house and into the barn. "DON'T TOUCH MY THINGS. THOSE ARE MY

THINGS. I NEED TO GO THROUGH IT," Hannah implored, her voice raw with shock and anger. The landlord stopped and glared at Hannah: "It's MY house. I pay the mortgage every month. Your lease ended. I even gave you $500 just to leave." As Hannah continued to pace frantically, the landlord approached me: "I've never seen anything like this." Through the front door, I saw the landlord's wife silhouetted in the doorframe, pushing a snow shovel through piles of the couple's possessions. The landlord practically spit the words at me, "She's sick. She's a hoarder. Like the show."

*   *   *

Time has not softened the sharp edge of this memory from 2014, five years into my study of families experiencing homelessness and its aftermath in rural Vermont and New Hampshire. This moment crystallizes the thorny tangle of poverty, mental illness, and substance use that appeared again and again over the years, enveloping families and stymying the neatness of analytic categories. As an anthropologist of mental health, this work is a departure in some ways from my previous close attention to the meanings and experiences of specific forms of mental illness and treatments. This work has taken me deep into the lives of families surviving at the margins of privilege in rural and small-town New England.

Ethnographic Setting: The Upper Valley

The Upper Connecticut River Valley—known locally as the Upper Valley—forms the border between central Vermont and central New Hampshire. This region, where I have lived and worked for more than 10 years, is covered by dense forest that yields to hayfields and pastureland. Each state is cleaved by a north-south highway that carries logging and milk trucks, commuters from distant towns to the region's main employers, and, on weekends, a steady stream of cars bearing New York and Massachusetts license plates zooming north to the mountains. Branching off these two main corridors is a network of smaller roads that link the region's small towns and villages. The wealthier Upper Valley towns bear a strong resemblance to notions of the "rural idyll" (Cloke et al., 2000)—vibrant places verging on postcard perfection. An epicenter of privilege surrounds Dartmouth College in the towns of Hanover, New Hampshire, and Norwich, Vermont—adjacent neighbors spanning the Connecticut River. These towns exemplify a nostalgic image of a "quintessential" New England: elegantly restored Colonial-era homes, towering elms, white-steepled churches. The sense of a "rural idyll" was captured in a 2014 *Yankee* magazine article that described the Upper Valley as "a collection of little-known small towns featuring the New England we all look for. You'll find beauty, nature, soft adventure, art—and even what *Forbes* magazine called, 'the best gelato in America'" (Tree, 2014). Yet the Upper Valley is a place of contrasts, with other towns worn by time and shifting economies. Unlike other rural environs in the South and Midwest, which have been more uniformly hard hit by shifts away from manufacturing and agricultural economies as well as boom-and-bust cycles of mineral extraction, the settings in which this ethnography takes place are a peculiar confluence of deep poverty and extraordinary privilege.

The Upper Valley is home to an Ivy League college, an academic medical center, and high-tech engineering companies that attract highly educated and skilled workers to the region. According to recent U.S. Census estimates, Hanover, New Hampshire, the town in which Dartmouth College is located, has a median household income of $103,558, and the median value of owner-occupied homes is $576,700 (U.S. Census Bureau, 2019). Less than 10 miles away is the town of Hartford, Vermont, where many of the families that I have worked with live. In Hartford, according to recent Census estimates, the median household income is substantially less than that of Hanover ($62,317), as are home values, with a median value of $227,000 (U.S. Census Bureau, 2020a). Although unemployment in the region is low—unlike in many rural areas of the country—the job opportunities for those with lower levels of education are limited to the low-wage service sector.

Microgeographies of Privilege and Poverty in Rural New England

Community discourses around these contrasts reveal what anthropologist Sherry Ortner (1998) has described as the "hidden life of class" in the United States and what I have come to think of as *microgeographies of privilege and poverty*, by which I mean the invisible borders that demarcate areas of immense wealth from towns with greater economic diversity. These microgeographies produce subtle yet insidious forms of social exclusion and paradoxical community responses to vulnerability. Deep traditions of philanthropy and progressive politics exist alongside efforts to limit affordable housing developments.[1] The discourse of community opposition expressed during town meetings and unfolding on the pages of the local newspapers does not explicitly make reference to social class. Instead, these efforts invoke discourses of rurality, whether linked to concerns over land conservation or cloaked in preservation of the "rural character" of pictur-esque small towns. "Rural character," as deployed in this debate, makes use of a particular imagining of *rural culture* that includes restored antique houses, general stores that boast "If we don't have it, you don't need it!," and organic community-supported agriculture (CSA) but erases the trailer homes, Dollar General and Walmart, and the dairy farmers forced by eco-nomic circumstances to sell their herds, with sometimes catastrophic men-tal health consequences.

The desperation of poverty is hidden in the Upper Valley, muted by the natural beauty of its landscape and hushed by the pride of its vulnerable people. Wealth, too, is downplayed by Yankee pragmatism, which favors Subarus over BMWs. With the extremes of poverty and wealth so masked, the reality and experience of housing insecurity are often obscured.

Ethnographic Entanglements over Time

The hidden nature of rural homelessness is what initially brought me to this work. My desire to work with families experiencing homelessness was driven by my earlier engagements with families impacted by childhood mental illness (Carpenter-Song, 2009a, 2009b). In 2009, as a postdoctoral researcher, I was eager to begin a new project, and I wrote a proposal at the suggestion of a colleague to study the lives of families experiencing home-lessness in Northern New England. Surveying the literature, it was clear that scant attention had been paid to housing insecurity in rural areas of the United States.[2] This piqued my interest to know more about families facing homelessness in rural communities. From the vantage point of 2020, these motivations strike me as anemic. What began as intellectual ques-tions have, in the crucible of time, been recast through entanglements with personal experience and moral grapplings. What I had originally conceived of as a 12-month project has now extended for more than a decade.

Work positioned on such a horizon of time invites both wonderings at the future and confrontations with the past, as the families and I have lived, grown, lost, and changed over 10 years. Over the course of this work, children were born; jobs were gained and lost; marriages were formed and

dissolved; and many, many moves were made. In witnessing and participating in this temporal flow, I have often thought of Byron Good's (1994)
notion of the "subjunctive mood" and Cheryl Mattingly's (1994) concept
of "emplotment" as families' experiences unfolded over many years. These
anthropological concepts, developed to describe qualities of illness narratives
(Good, 1994) and therapeutic work (Mattingly, 1994), foreground the nonlinear and unpredictable as key dimensions of how people experience and
make meaning of events, actions, and motivations. As Mattingly (1994) has
written:

> If lived experience positions us in a fluid space between a past and a future, then
> what we experience is strongly marked by the possible. Meaning itself, from this
> perspective, is always in suspense. If the meaning of the present, and even of the
> past, is contingent on what unfolds in the future, then what is happening and
> what has happened is not a matter of facts but of interpretive possibilities which
> are vulnerable to an unknown future. (p. 820)

At junctures during this work, when I was confronted with the question of
whether to continue the research,[3] I felt an acute sense of that "unknown
future" in the tug of indeterminacy—the desire to know how families fared
over time and the keen awareness that such understanding would always
remain stubbornly partial.

Longitudinal research approaches have been noted as particularly important for research on homelessness as a way to contextualize experiences of
homelessness and, thus, to avoid medicalizing social and political problems
(Biederman & Lindsey, 2014; Snow, Anderson, & Koegel, 1994). The long
view of families' experiences has destabilized the category of "homelessness" (cf. Hopper, 2003) as I witnessed families oscillate between periods of
relative security, instability, and crisis. Engagement over time has revealed
radically divergent trajectories in the cohort of families, with some being
"shattered" and others coming to occupy a fragile security. Longitudinal
research illuminates the reciprocal production of lived experience and
social-institutional inequalities (Jenkins, 2015b; Jenkins & Csordas, 2020)
in the context of everyday efforts to imagine and work toward "possible
selves" (Parish, 2008) and to "have a life" (Jenkins and Csordas, 2020).

The view from 10 years out also forces me to confront an uncomfortable
fact of my positionality as my own trajectory has been one of increasing
security over time while documenting deep struggle and, in some cases, devastation among my interlocuters. At the start of the project, my positioning

had more in common with the families—insecure, temporary employment, modest salary, and unpredictable housing[4] as I commuted to Dartmouth a few days a week from Rhode Island, where I lived with my husband, who was then finishing his graduate studies. I am not drawing an equivalence between my experience and theirs. I was highly educated, pursuing work that I found meaningful at an Ivy League institution, and not yet a parent at the beginning of the research. Yet the mobility and insecurity that I experienced in the early years of this work provided me a limited experiential point of departure[5] for understanding the impact of moving between housing settings and the challenges of sustaining connections amid mobility.

Methods

Beginning in the fall of 2009, I conducted ethnographic visits with families that I recruited through a partnership with a Vermont-based shelter I call Safe Harbor. In a twist of good fortune and serendipity, the executive director of the shelter took a chance on me and welcomed me into the setting. Two shelter staff members were instrumental in making connections to families, taking time during their busy days to explain the study to those in residence at the shelter and to make introductions. To be eligible for the study, adults were currently without housing and were parents of dependent children. Both single- and two-parent households were eligible for inclusion in the study. The shelter had capacity to house eight families; of these, six families initially agreed to participate in the research. One young mother fell out of contact early in the study in the fall of 2009 following the birth of her second child. Five families continued in the study. Study procedures were approved by the Dartmouth College Committee for the Protection of Human Subjects (#21748), and participants gave consent and assent to participate in the study. All participant names in this book are pseudonyms. To recognize the time and effort that families generously gave in inviting me into the intimate realms of their experience, families received a modest research stipend of $50 per month for participating in the study.[6]

As Judith Marti (2016) has noted in her description of "studying at home": "Just because one's field site is close by does not mean it's accessible, that the doors will fly open" (p. 15). I am deeply grateful both for the willingness of Safe Harbor staff members to facilitate my connections to residents of the shelter and, most especially, for the families' courage in inviting me into their lives as a witness and confidante. From that initial point of entry—a leap of faith on the part of families—I worked hard to prove myself worthy of the gift of access to lived experiences of profound vulnerability. This involved communicating the peculiar role of the ethnographer as I explained to families that I hoped to learn about their lives and their experiences of homelessness by spending time with them. They graciously accepted these terms with the understanding that I, in turn, would endeavor to share their experiences to deepen awareness of rural homelessness and to advocate for changes within practice and policy to improve the lives of families experiencing housing insecurity.[7] In these efforts as an engaged scholar, I am guided by models of "accompaniment" (Farmer, 2013; Watkins, 2015) and have aimed to disrupt traditional research hierarchies while also acknowledging my privilege as an ethnographer. Trust was built over time through my efforts to be a reliable presence—someone who would show up (and keep showing up)—and to embody a stance of openness and nonjudgment toward their experiences.

Over the course of the study, from its beginnings in 2009 to this writing in 2021, I have conducted over 320 scheduled ethnographic visits[8] with families. With my engagements with families forming the centerpiece of the research, this work has been augmented over the years with interviews with healthcare and social service providers, interviews and focus groups with a broader group of individuals with lived experiences of housing insecurity, and participatory research approaches conducted in collaboration with individuals with lived experience and care providers. I layer insights from these multiple research encounters throughout the book to offer a greater diversity of perspectives grounded in lived experience of housing insecurity, mental health and substance use, and the voices of those striving to care for marginalized families in rural communities.

During ethnographic visits with families, I occupied the dual role of participant and observer, striving to immerse myself in the settings and interactions of family life, sharing in their everyday lives while also remaining an "outsider" attentive to the aims of the research (Emerson, Fretz, & Shaw, 2011; Marti, 2016; Spradley, 1980/2016). Mirroring the mobility induced by chronic housing insecurity, the research was conducted as mobile anthropology (Jenkins, 2015b) across a range of community, clinical, and social service settings. The approach I used has also been described as "problem-oriented" ethnography—research that is focused on particular challenges and experiences that "transcend the boundaries of locality" (Jenkins & Csordas, 2020, p. 24). In this case, the research was initially oriented toward the problem of homelessness. Over time, this scope expanded to include broader experiences of poverty and housing insecurity as well as the experiences of families as they navigated through the rural landscape of care. The settings and activities of the visits were intended to reflect their usual habits and routines. Activities during ethnographic visits were guided by the families and centered on domestic chores, running errands, and simply spending time together. Over time, this strategy has yielded knowledge of the "rhythms of daily life" (Jenkins, 1997, p. 23) for each family.

Ethnographic visits blended observations of settings and interactions with informal interviews. Over the course of the study, I also conducted focused, in-depth interviews with parents. Field notes were taken following each ethnographic visit to systematically document the settings, activities, and dialogue that occurred during the visit (Emerson et al., 2011). Interviews were digitally audio-recorded and transcribed. The act of writing field notes is recognized as an interpretive process and, as such, is a foundational aspect of data analysis (Emerson et al., 2011). My analytic strategy was inductive and focused on developing salient and prominent themes (Braun & Clarke, 2006). Field notes and transcripts were archived chronologically by family. I conducted ongoing immersive reviews of the data and used Scrivener to organize text excerpts by topic/concept. I subsequently reviewed aggregated data and used memo-ing as a technique to construct thematic insights (Padgett, 2012).

Family Characteristics

At the heart of this book are the experiences of five families that I grew to know over many years. Woven throughout are the experiences of Jim and Hannah, a couple in their 40s with four children; Abigail and Nancy, two single mothers in their late teens and 20s, respectively, who were raising toddler-age daughters when we met; Tara, a mother in her 20s who had a young son when we met and an on-again-off-again relationship with her husband; and Barbara, a woman in her 40s who was raising two teenagers and had a long-term boyfriend. Over time, some families grew: Abigail went on to have two more children, both boys; Nancy had a son; and Tara gave birth to a daughter. Other families experienced losses. Jim and Hannah as well as Tara had their children taken into state custody. Relationships changed over time, too. Nancy married and later divorced, Tara divorced, and Abigail was involved in a series of relationships over the course of the study.

In all families except one, I engaged with women as my primary interlocuters. In the other instance, both the husband and wife were deeply involved in the study. All adults in the study self-identified as White and non-Hispanic. Of the five women, four had completed high school, and two had some college credits; the male participant had a bachelor's degree. The average household income among participating families was $856 per month, including wages, cash benefits, and food stamps. Out-of-pocket housing costs for participating families averaged $478 per month.[9] The average market rent of the apartments or houses for participants was $1,002 per month; two families had Section 8 vouchers. With respect to adult participants' health status, many were seriously burdened by numerous chronic physical and mental health conditions. All but one adult participant self-reported having at least one psychiatric disorder, including depression ($n=4$), anxiety ($n=3$), bipolar disorder ($n=1$), attention-deficit hyperactivity disorder (ADHD) ($n=2$), post-traumatic stress disorder (PTSD) ($n=2$), and traumatic brain injury ($n=1$).

An Anthropology of the Intimate

My ethnographic engagements were informed by a meaning-centered, experienced-based anthropological theoretical framework (Good, 1994; Jenkins, 2015a; Kleinman, 1988). Experience-based approaches aim to elicit the meanings of personal and cultural phenomena from the first-person perspectives of participants such that "the basic units of analysis are established by the people we study rather than by the anthropologist as alien observer" (Bruner, 1986, p. 9). As more recent articulations of experience-based approaches make clear, attention to lived experience also demands interrogation of the impress of political, economic, and social structures (Biehl et al., 2007; Jenkins, 2015b; Jenkins & Csordas, 2020). Grounded in deep immersion with our interlocuters, ethnography illuminates the filaments of connection between lived experience and structural forces. By tacking between the messiness of lives and the broader structures and systems, experience-based approaches open opportunities to bring into view constraining forces alongside the tangible manifestations of agency in people's everyday efforts and actions.

Methodologically, this work aligns with person-centered ethnography (LeVine, 1982; Levy & Hollan, 2015). Person-centered ethnographic approaches foreground "the point of view of the acting, intending, and attentive subject" and "actively explore the emotional saliency and motivational force of cultural beliefs, symbols, and structures, rather than to assume such salience and force" (Levy & Hollan, 2015, p. 313). Building on person-centered approaches, I conceptualize this research as family-centered ethnography (Shohet & Anderson, 2017). A theoretical through line from my previous work reveals itself as I advance the family as an ethnographic site for the enlivenment of concepts of intersubjectivity—the family as crucible for the creation and blurring of selves—and, following others (e.g., Mattingly, 2014), for the enactment and production of moral experience (Kleinman, 1998, 2007). I conceptualize the form of ethnographic engagement on which this book is based as *an anthropology of the intimate*. Anthropological methods have been described as a "science of intimacy, of intimate connections" (Kelly, 2014; see also Myers, 2015, 2016). Indeed, ethnography is intimate by design. Yet, too often, the hallmark intimacy of ethnographic fieldwork is obscured or tamed by the abstractions of anthropological theorizing. As Michael Jackson (2013) states of the distrust of matters of subjectivity in anthropology:

> In the establishment of anthropology as a science of the social or cultural, entire domains of human experience were occluded or assigned to other disciplines, most notably the lived body, the life of the senses, ethics and imagination, the emotions, materiality, and technology. Subjectivity was conflated with roles, rules, routines, and rituals. Individual variations were seen as deviations from the norm. Contingency was played down. Collective representations determined the real. . . . As such, persons were depicted one-dimensionally, their lives little more than allegories and instantiations of politics, historical, or social processes. (p. 4)

In contrast to traditional anthropological approaches, close engagement with families over time plunges the ethnographer into intimate realms of human experience, demanding attention to complexities, contingencies, and paradoxes of care (cf. Garcia, 2008; Mattingly, 2010). This book stays intentionally close to the experiences of families. The intimacy of working closely with families over time yields a unique understanding of rural poverty and its consequences for the mental health and well-being of families as they endure, and struggle against, threats to their survival.

Marginalization in Rural New England

It is crucial to recognize that although all of the parents[10] with whom I engaged were White and non-Hispanic, homelessness disproportionately impacts Black/African American and Indigenous populations in the United States. Legacies of dispossession and endemic structural racism in housing policies are reflected in findings that 39% of all people experiencing homelessness in the United States in 2020 were Black/African American despite representing 12% of the U.S. population and that Indigenous people accounted for 5% of the homeless population in 2020 while being 1% of the U.S. population (Henry et al., 2020). By contrast, 48% of all people experiencing homelessness in the U.S. in 2020 were White while being 74% of the total U.S. population (Henry et al., 2020).

At this moment of national reckoning on insidious forms of racism and the stubborn persistence of racial inequities, a focus on White families experiencing homelessness may appear to elide these realities. However, the focus of this work on homelessness in rural U.S. communities partially explains the demographic makeup of participating families. Black/White inequities in homelessness are least pronounced in rural areas, with White people accounting for 71% of people experiencing homelessness while being 84% of the rural population (Moses, 2019). In addition, the families that engaged in the study are broadly representative of the demographics in Northern New England. In Vermont and New Hampshire 92.6% and 89.8%, respectively, of the total state population identifies as White and non-Hispanic (U.S. Census, 2020b).

bell hooks (2000) has written that "poor white folks" constitute the "hidden face of poverty" in the United States (p. 117). Those experiencing homelessness in rural U.S. communities have been described as America's "lost nation" (Craft-Rosenberg et al., 2000, p. 863). More recently, there has been increased attention to rural White populations in the wake of the rise of the Tea Party and Trumpism (Hochschild, 2016) as well as the notable decrease in life expectancy among non–college-educated Whites linked to so-called deaths of despair (Case & Deaton, 2020). The circumstances of the families in this research track with the broad sociopolitical forces constraining opportunities for those with lower levels of education. In this way, though this research focuses on marginalization in Northern New England, the experiences of intense struggle detailed in this book illuminate broader social and cultural realities within the contemporary U.S. while recognizing the limits of the research to engage with all of the complexities of race, poverty, and homelessness in the United States.

Goals of the Book

In this book, I aim to take readers into experiences that often remain hidden. With families as my focus, this work has involved crossing over intimate thresholds to enter into the physical and interactive spaces of family life and to become attuned to the affective flows of daily experience. I experience this work as a form of intense paying attention, resonating with Spradley's notion of "explicit awareness" in ethnographic research (2016, p. 55). My senses heighten to become aware of subtleties of expression, shifts in tone of voice, details of a room and its contents, and odors and textures surrounding me. This is work done at kitchen tables and on rickety porches. I'm privy to shifts in self-presentation as my interlocutors move between public and private spaces. I witness the shedding of niceties and the softening of hard edges, flashes of anger, the fog of boredom, and the creeping shadows of sadness. I see parental love manifest in eyes shadowed by dark circles, the bodily markers of a sleepless night spent caring for a sick child. I am taken into worlds that usually remain hidden—crusty dishes stacked precariously in a kitchen sink, framed photographs of smiling faces, the sting of Pine-Sol wafting from a just-mopped floor, cigarette butts piled in an ashtray.

Grounded in the intimacy of close attention to family life, I explore families' entanglements with the institutions and services that are intended to support their health and survival. With a small cohort of families as the methodological and conceptual grounding for this work, I have also engaged with a range of others occupying positions in the rural landscape of care, including shelter-based case managers, mental health providers, attorneys, and leaders within social services and health systems.

Families experiencing homelessness and housing insecurity move through a kaleidoscopic landscape of housing and social services, health care, mental health and substance use services, legal services, and the child welfare system. And yet, despite being caught in the "psychiatric net" (Carpenter-Song, 2009a, p. 81) and a great many other service "nets," most of the families remained quite tenuously and ineffectively engaged with these professional services and seemed instead to slip through the spaces in-between. In exploring the complex and often ineffective intersection between marginalized families and care providers, I focus on the missed opportunities and unintended consequences of engagement with "helping" organizations.

The frame of missed opportunities and unintended consequences offers an interpretive space that engages with the tensions at play within institutions of care. Following others (Good, 1994), I have found Foucauldian applications of the medical gaze (Foucault, 1994) to be overly deterministic and at odds with the orientation toward care I find among most who work in health and social services. Likewise, traditional critiques of biomedicine within medical anthropology do not adequately engage with the complexity of the lived experience of trying to care for others day in and day out. Yet this moral sensibility, often articulated simply as wanting to "help others" or to "be of service," is not, in itself, sufficient to guard against negative experiences or poor outcomes. I explore these tensions throughout the book to raise questions, identify missed opportunities to support marginalized families, and consider possibilities for meaningful recovery.

The book is organized to first ground readers in the lived experiences of families surviving in poverty before moving to consider the landscape of care for marginalized families within rural New England.

Chapter 2, "Becoming Homeless in Rural New England," details the precipitants of homelessness for the families in the study, highlighting the specific challenges of being poor in rural and small-town New England communities. The chapter aims to highlight the ways in which lived experiences of extreme poverty are grounded in and shaped by cultural context. Just as rural America is not monolithic, neither are the experiences of homelessness. The chapter immerses the reader in daily life in the family shelter, a place I call Safe Harbor, and describes families' efforts to search for affordable housing. This chapter also introduces Donna Friedman's (2000) concept of "parenting in public," which I borrow to describe the forms of surveillance enacted by helping organizations. Even in a context that strives to be family centered, parents still found that activities of daily life—from housekeeping chores to money management to parenting styles—were subject to monitoring and regulation by shelter staff. This theme will be picked up on and elaborated on in subsequent chapters. This chapter concludes with a discussion of the moral valences as well as the personal and cultural meanings of homelessness in the Northern New England context.

Chapter 3, "Life on the Edge," introduces the concept of *fundamental insecurity*. This concept is intended to evoke the totality and pervasiveness of instability, impermanence, and mobility in the lives of rural families that have experienced homelessness. This definition links material conditions of poverty to social forms of precarity in rural New England. Existing studies of homeless families concentrate on the periods of time when families are literally homeless or living in shelters. The research on which is book is based is unique in examining family life during periods of homelessness as well as *after* being sheltered. Taking a long view of families' trajectories has allowed me to document what happens to families in the community following a period of homelessness. This chapter highlights a key finding: homelessness is episodic, but housing insecurity is chronic, with families continuing to exist "on the edge" of homelessness. This chapter explores the precarity and resourcefulness of "life on the edge" by examining chronic housing insecurity, low-wage work, precarious relationships, and efforts to "make it" in rural New England.

Chapter 4, "Paradoxes of Care," examines the complex and often ineffective intersection between marginalized families and the systems of care intended to support families. Despite struggling with chronic health, mental health, and substance use challenges in the context of living in poverty, over time it became clear that most families remained quite tenuously and haphazardly engaged with professional services—a phenomenon I term *paradoxes of care*. This chapter describes three patterns of paradoxes of care: (1) on my terms, (2) going through the motions, and (3) grasping at straws. Paradoxes of care highlight the missed opportunities and unintended consequences of engagement with "helping" organizations.

Chapter 5, "Shattered Families," builds on themes from the previous chapter to illuminate the high stakes involved in the misalignment of the experiences of marginalized families and systems of care. Families in the study navigated through the rural landscape of care to meet their basic needs yet, in doing so, risked having their financial and housing insecurity call into question their adequacy as parents. For some, this had the tragic consequence of fundamentally refashioning supportive services into an apparatus of surveillance and harm. I detail the experiences of two families to critically examine the gradual unraveling of life in the wake of losing custody of their children and to identify points of entry for disrupting trajectories of devastation.

Chapter 6, "Toward Security Following Homelessness," examines the personal, social, and structural resources foundational to maintaining a semblance of security in the midst of precarity. I argue that it is the confluence of available structural supports and particular subjective orientations that create possibilities for greater security and opportunities for families to meaningfully engage with existing services and resources. There is a clear need to attend not only to the access and availability of services but also to subjective orientations that shape everyday efforts to survive, engagements with diverse forms of care, policies enabling affordable housing, opportunities for livable wages, and compassionate healthcare for all families.

A key aim of this research is to raise awareness of the challenges faced by families during periods of homelessness and during their efforts to rebuild their lives by identifying crucial inflection points that either support or erode possibilities for meaningful recovery at the intersection of poverty, mental illness, and substance use. As a medical and psychological anthropologist, I am deeply committed to engaged scholarship and have aimed throughout my career to work across disciplinary boundaries in order to render anthropological insights relevant to broader audiences of clinicians, public health and health services researchers, and policymakers. In these efforts, I endeavor to position myself as an "accompanier" (Farmer, 2013; Watkins, 2015), articulating possibilities for reimagining policies and care grounded in the lived experiences of those with whom I have had the privilege to work. I approach this work with humility and in collaboration and solidarity with families experiencing poverty, mental illness, and substance use:

> Interventions are not to be proposed "from the outside," but determined with participants, alongside, through dialogue and critical reflection. The accompanier needs to be a reliable presence, making consistent and respectful visits, or living alongside. Through their openness to dialogue, the needs of individuals and of the community emerge and can be engaged together in a respectful and thoughtful manner. (Watkins, 2015, p. 329)

To that end and in that spirit, in the conclusion, I distill key lessons that can be drawn from families' experiences to inform practice, service provision, and advocacy with and for marginalized families in rural communities.

2 Becoming Homeless in Rural New England

"There are homeless people here?"

At the start of this work in 2009, when I told friends and colleagues about my new project focused on rural homelessness, they often paused, tightened their brows, and asked, "There are homeless people here?"

Families experiencing homelessness have been described as "America's lost nation" (Craft-Rosenberg et al., 2000, p. 863), and this invisibility is compounded by the hidden nature of housing insecurity in the rural United States.[1] Janet Fitchen's (1992) work on poverty and homelessness in upstate New York in the 1980s identified several distinguishing features of rural homelessness. Those who become homeless in rural areas may live in their cars, sleep in the woods, or find shelter in abandoned buildings (Fitchen, 1992). In rural communities, many surviving in poverty double up with friends and family, stay in motels, or live in substandard housing (Butler, 1997; Fitchen, 1992). The limited evidence suggests that, compared with urban homeless populations, rural homeless populations are younger, more highly educated, less likely to have disabilities, more likely to have been employed or to be currently employed, and more likely to be women with children (First et al., 1994; Nord and Luloff, 1995).

In his landmark research tracing homelessness in New York City, anthropologist Kim Hopper (2003) offers a searing description of urban homelessness:

> the half-naked man cavorting in the steam pouring out of vents at a street construction site early one morning, wraithlike in the glow of mercury-vapor lights; the sobbing figure of a woman sitting on the stone steps of a church, the still body of a man lying prone on the sidewalk, the plaintive importuning of a beggar at the subway turnstile—each studiously ignored by passersby. (p. 3)

Such images are incongruous with daily experiences in the small towns of the Upper Valley. Anyone walking through these villages will not encounter people crouched against the elements in doorways or sleeping on the sidewalk. Encampments of unhoused people do exist in this setting but are largely out of sight. Unlike the "city's forsaken" described by Hopper (2003, p. 3), none of the families I first met in the fall of 2009 at a shelter in central Vermont had lived "on the street" or "slept rough" in the outdoors with their children. Theirs was not a public homelessness but instead one lived on couches and doubled up in apartments, with nights spent in cars and stretches spent in seedy pay-by-the-week motels. If a primary feature of urban homelessness is its visibility, homelessness in rural areas is largely hidden, accounting, in part, for the question I encountered so frequently in my early work.[2]

The difficulty of documenting people living in remote areas or doubling up obscures the extent of housing problems in rural settings. Rural homeless advocates caution against viewing statistics on homelessness as a precise measurement, noting that these figures underestimate the number of people who are precariously housed in rural settings. A few months into the study, the challenge of documenting rural homeless populations was put into bold relief for me in an email exchange I had with the director of homeless outreach at a social service organization in New Hampshire. After taking a look at the data available from the National Alliance to End Homelessness, I was curious to hear the director's take on the statistics. I wondered if the reported numbers reflected what she saw on a day-to-day basis in her community-based work. I asked if she could provide me with more local data on the rate of homelessness in the Upper Valley region. In the email response I received back from her, she noted the challenges of a precise measurement of the population experiencing homelessness in rural areas:

> Problems with measuring rural homelessness is this—you are dealing with "doubled up dependent" or "couch surfers." [There are] people so remote they don't access services so they don't get counted. Those are just two of the barriers. We do a "point in time" count once a year where we count the homeless encounters we have in a 24-hour period. but that tells us nothing. What if that was the 24 hours someone was in the ER sleeping or didn't have minutes on their cell to call us? . . . I wish I could be more help. (personal communication, February 11, 2010)

As her response illustrates, accurately measuring the scale of homelessness in rural areas is hindered by features of rural geography and by the manifestations of rural housing insecurity.

Although imperfect, the annual Point-in-Time (PIT) counts offer a proxy of the scope of homelessness. The PIT is a national effort by the U.S. Department of Housing and Urban Development (HUD) conducted annually to count the number of sheltered and unsheltered people experiencing homelessness on a single night in January. During these efforts, local housing advocates and volunteers tally all the people experiencing homelessness they encounter in a 24-hour period, including those in often out-of-the-way places in small rural towns—shelter settings, the parking lot of Walmart after dark, and the encampments behind strip malls and beneath highway overpasses.

In 2009, the year the study began, the PIT reported the total homeless population in Vermont as 1,214 and reported 193 households with children experiencing homelessness (HUD, 2021). In New Hampshire in 2009, the PIT reported the total homeless population as 1,645 and reported 259 households with children experiencing homelessness (HUD, 2021). The available data indicate that there were increases in the overall homeless population in Vermont and New Hampshire during the early years of the study. Tracking with the fallout from the financial crisis in 2008, estimates from Vermont show that the homeless population increased more than 27% between 2008 and 2009 (Sermons & Witte, 2011). According to the Bureau of Homeless and Housing Services, New Hampshire's homeless population increased by 18% between 2010 and 2011 (*Union Leader*, March 30, 2011). The number of families experiencing homelessness in the region also increased. Whereas "homeless families were virtually unheard of in earlier eras" (Bassuk, 1993, p. 337), families now constitute the "new face" of homelessness. Available data indicate that the number of families experiencing homelessness in Vermont increased by more than 59% between 2008 and 2009 (Sermons & Witte, 2011); New Hampshire experienced a 30% increase in homeless families between 2010 and 2011 (*Union Leader*, March 30, 2011).

More recent data suggest a mixed picture of homelessness in the region. Point-in-Time counts from the Vermont Coalition to End Homelessness and the Chittenden County Homeless Alliance reported a 16% decrease from 2018 to 2019 for individuals experiencing homelessness but found that chronically homeless households increased by 12% (Vermont Coalition to End Homelessness, 2020). The PIT in Vermont in 2020 reported the total homeless population as 1,110 and reported 124 households with children experiencing homelessness, decreases from the beginning of the study in

2009. In New Hampshire, overall homelessness increased by 10%, and the number of people in families experiencing homelessness increased by 14% between 2016 and 2018 (New Hampshire Coalition to End Homelessness, 2018). The PIT in New Hampshire in 2020 reported the total homeless population as 1,675 (HUD, 2021), a slight increase from the beginning of the study in 2009. The number of households with children experiencing homelessness reported in the New Hampshire PIT in 2020 was 219 (HUD, 2021), a decrease from the number reported in 2009. More recent data from 2020 indicate increases in homelessness in the wake of the COVID-19 pandemic (Elletson, 2020).[3]

Efforts to count homeless individuals likely underestimate the extent of homelessness. Some individuals are so remote that they do not access services and therefore are not always known to local advocacy and resource organizations. PIT counts also provide little insight into those precariously housed and living on the edge of homelessness. Further complicating and obscuring the issue, defining homelessness has been a "fundamental and persistent problem" (Amore et al., 2011, p. 20). Efforts to categorize homelessness, such as the European Typology of Homelessness and Housing Exclusion (ETHOS), articulate a range of settings and situations that variously constitute homelessness and insecure housing. While such typologies may be useful for directing attention and resources to relatively more severe situations, some researchers have critiqued the "seemingly arbitrary threshold between homelessness and housing insecurity" (Amore et al., 2011, p. 25). This threshold may be even more problematic in the context of rural settings. As Cloke and colleagues (Cloke et al., 2000) have noted, definitions of homelessness tend to focus on rooflessness, which does not take into account varied and complex housing "mobilities" in rural areas (Cloke et al., 2003; see also Meert & Bourgeois, 2005). This is reflected in how homelessness is officially defined by the U.S. Stewart B. McKinney Homeless Assistance Act, which emphasizes the total lack of a fixed residence. In contrast, scholarly conceptualizations of homelessness in rural areas emphasize housing instability (Fitchen, 1991; Patton, 1998). Yvonne Vissing (1996) suggests that "housing distress" or "displaced persons" are better terms to describe the day-to-day experiences of rural homeless populations. Following from this, individuals and families that become homeless are not a distinct "poor apart" (Hopper, 1991, p. 758, 2003). As Rob Whitley (2013) has argued, categorical distinctions between the rural homeless and rural poor people may be spurious. Homelessness as a broad category obscures the diversity of circumstances and strategies employed by those surviving in poverty to secure housing. It is the case that some in this rural setting are unhoused and live in tents and other makeshift forms of shelter. Such experiences are not emblematic of the families described in this book. My focus on families likely compounds the hidden nature of rural housing precarity as families go to great lengths to avoid literal homelessness. As I detail in these pages, however, such efforts often entail high mobility and the ever-present threat of housing loss.

The experiences of families contending with housing insecurity in rural areas are also obscured by particular imaginings of "homelessness" and "the rural." Paul Cloke and his colleagues (2000) working in the United Kingdom, have described the "conceptual noncoupling" (p. 727) of rurality and homelessness, arguing that romantic conceptions of the "rural idyll" (p. 721) inhibit engagement with poverty and displacement in these settings. It is important to contextualize this argument within the cultural context of the United Kingdom, where deeply classed notions of the rural idyll are tied to the collective imagination of the English countryside and landed gentry.

As I consider the relevance of Cloke and his colleagues' (2000) conceptual noncoupling to rural New England, two points emerge. First, as described in chapter 1, the ethnographic setting is marked by extremes of wealth and poverty. Yet this is not the only form of conceptual noncoupling. The second draws on a distinctly American set of orientations to "the rural." Such renderings of rurality often cement an association of rural with poor.[4] However, I would argue that the rural poor are imagined as rooted in ramshackle houses and dilapidated trailers nestled in dark mountainous hollows or perched on desolate farmland. This serves to decouple the association with homelessness though the presumption that, however humble, housing is accessible and cheap in rural towns.

Public awareness of the shortage of affordable housing as a key social justice and ethical challenge in the United States has grown (see, e.g., Desmond, 2016). But again, attention to this urgent issue has primarily centered on urban areas, with the emerging tent cities on the West Coast and bodies heaped on New York sidewalks fitting a cultural logic and narrative of dystopian fallout of the capitalist icons of Silicon Valley and Wall Street. Yet in the valley where I live and work far from these urban centers with runaway real estate valuations, families also face deep challenges accessing affordable housing. The cost of living, although lower than in major metropolitan areas, remains high. In Windsor County, Vermont, where most study participants resided, the fair market rent for a two-bedroom unit in 2020 was $1,018 per month (National Low Income Housing Coalition, 2020). To be considered affordable (i.e., a dwelling that a household can obtain for not more than 30% of its income), these units would require an hourly wage of $19.58, and yet the state minimum wage was only $10.96 (National Low Income Housing Coalition, 2020). In Windsor County, 22% of renters spent 30% to 49% of their income on housing, and 25% of renters spent 50% or more of their income on housing (Vermont Housing Finance Agency, 2018). As elsewhere in the United States (Desmond, 2016), most low-income households in Vermont do not receive housing assistance (Center on Budget and Policy Priorities, 2019; Vermont Housing Finance Agency, 2012). The shortage of affordable housing was felt acutely by families in the study, each of whom searched for months to find housing in order to exit the shelter.

Pathways into Homelessness

Understanding what brings a family into a place like Safe Harbor and what circumstances surround a housing crisis serves as a point of departure for engaging with the experiences of families living in poverty in rural New England. As noted above, in rural communities, there is no strict separation between families surviving on the economic margins and those experiencing homelessness (Whitley, 2013). These are phenomena that exist along a porous boundary, with families oscillating between periods of relative stability and instability. When I first met the families in this study, all were living in the aftermath of a housing crisis that had eventually brought them into the shelter setting at Safe Harbor.

The specific circumstances surrounding a family's housing crisis varied, but over the years, I came to recognize common catalysts of homelessness across the individuals and families I grew to know at Safe Harbor—undergoing a separation or divorce, experiencing domestic violence, losing a job, getting sick, exacerbating mental health issues and substance use, or simply trying to bridge the gap between low wages and high rents in the area. Homelessness in rural areas has been linked to structural factors, including worsening rural poverty, a lack of affordable housing, and increases in single-parent households (Butler, 1997; Fitchen, 1991). In a study of family homelessness in rural Ohio funded by the National Institute of Mental Health (NIMH), Richard First, John Rife, and Beverly Toomey (1994) found that almost half of the families experienced economic factors (including unemployment, difficulty paying rent, and eviction) and that a third of the families cited personal problems (including conflict and dissolution of relationships) as the cause of their becoming homeless.

These findings resonated with the experiences of those staying at Safe Harbor. During a focus group, residents in the family shelter shared what had led them to become homeless. Kate described escaping an abusive relationship:

> It was pretty verbally abusive—a relationship where, you know, anything I did was wrong and, you know, awful. Every fight we got into, he'd always tell me to get out of his house. And it never felt like a home. [She describes a conflict between her husband and her mother.] It's a long, very long story. And he had asked me to leave his home. And at that point in time, I decided, "That's it. I'm done." I chose to leave. It was on a Friday, and, um, I called [Safe Harbor] on a Saturday, and I was able to get in by Wednesday.

Another resident nodded her head as Kate shared her experience and then revealed that she, too, had experienced domestic violence and had come to Safe Harbor because "the only family that I have is gone." Others had lost jobs and quickly ran out of money, as Caleb described:

> We both lost our jobs in the winter and things have kinda fallen apart from there. Um, we went broke in about a month. We went through all our reserves, and then that was it. We lost our apartment, and we ended up living in our van for about three weeks in January. And then we went to motels. The state helped us pay for 'em. And then we got in here [the shelter].

For Faith, low-wage work was insufficient to cover the cost of rent in the area:

> I worked, and I just couldn't pay for rent. I tapped out all my resources for it—the state, other community outreach projects. We just couldn't afford it. And the landlord let us stay as long as he could afford to let us stay, and, um, we just couldn't do it and ended up having to let him evict us. And I called here, and they put me down on the waiting list. And she called me two days later. She had a room for us!

Echoing these residents' experiences, the director of Safe Harbor shared her perspectives on the primary contributors to becoming homeless:

> I think our profile [at the shelter] fits the national profile that identifies inadequate income or loss of income, unaffordable housing, and lack of—insufficient supply of—affordable housing; domestic violence situations that break up households and cause people who may have been getting by economically and emotionally

to be getting by on neither domain; medical health and mental health issues as another category. And then the other category is natural disaster, whether it is fire or flood or whatever the cause is—a disruption in available resources for a household. And I would say that we see most people who are homeless having some combination of those elements as part of the picture.

A shortage of affordable housing in the Upper Valley was a primary structural condition contributing to families' vulnerability to housing crises. In interviews with staff at Safe Harbor, all immediately identified the lack of affordable housing as a key challenge facing the individuals and families they serve. Amy, who worked the night shift at the family shelter, put it in stark terms: "Incredibly high rent. This area is like low-, low-paying jobs, and rent is crazy. . . . It's really really horrid what they can charge for rent up here." Jamie, a case manager who had been at Safe Harbor since its beginnings in the 1980s, reflected on the local housing situation:

There's really not a lot of good answers out there for people. Because you really need two incomes, and often with two incomes at [a grocery store] or something, it's *still* not enough to pay market rent. And then the subsidized options are few and far between.

Compounding the challenge posed by the limited housing stock in the region, landlords were often unwilling to accept applicants with poor credit histories, especially in the context of the financial crisis of 2008, which formed a backdrop to the study in its early years. As Tara lamented, "You gotta have top-notch credit." Young adults in the study commonly noted that their lack of a rental history posed a barrier to obtaining housing. Even among families that had Section 8 or other subsidized housing vouchers, finding an apartment or a house to rent remained difficult in a rural setting marked by an extremely limited inventory of rental units and with few high-density housing communities.[5] In this context, landlords had the upper hand, and the scarcity of affordable housing put families at risk of accepting properties in substandard condition, with ensuing risks of injury from faulty wiring, lead paint, and mold in aging, dilapidated structures.

Health problems figured prominently in contributing to poverty and homelessness among many families, with lifetimes of poverty etched on their bodies. I would often find myself stunned to learn that the chronological age of someone I had met at the shelter was years (or decades) younger than their apparent age. When Tara's young son flashed his goofy grin, dark stains at the gumline were a bodily archive of the lead in the water pipes in their last apartment. It was the discovery of this environmental toxin that had landed them with "nowhere to go" and into the shelter. Unlike many of the families with deep roots in the area, Jim and Hannah had moved to New England only a few years before I met them. Prior to moving to New England from the South, Jim was injured in an accident and had difficulty accessing health services to treat his disability. This prompted the family to move in order to access healthcare for Jim and the couple's children, several of whom also lived with chronic health conditions. Their decision to move vaulted the family into uncharted territory and away from networks of kin and friends. When their finances "became a complete disaster" and they faced eviction, the couple had few options and moved the family into Safe Harbor.

Drugs were a part of the story for how some families came to be at the shelter. One afternoon, while I was meeting with Barbara over a cup of milky coffee at Dunkin' Donuts, she opened up about the time preceding her family's move into Safe Harbor. Barbara shared that after inheriting some money, she and her boyfriend had spiraled deeper and deeper into substance use:

> You know, I lost everything. I lost a lot of—everything I had. You know, selling it to be able to use and all kinds of stuff. And money, just—just thousands upon thousands of dollars that, you know, just got—that's what you did. That's who you hung around with—those kind of people that were just the lowest of the low. And you look around, and you couldn't even imagine that you'd found yourself in a situation like that. I mean, I could blow $1,000 in a night, Elizabeth. I know all about it. We went through $30,000 in a very short period of time.

She elaborated on her family's slide into poverty in the cycle of addiction:

> You sell your soul to the devil when you're into those things. The things that you do—you look back on, and you think of it, and you say, "I can't believe that I let myself go so low." You know what I mean? And in a sense of selling everything. Selling half the stuff that the kids had . . . trying to get enough money to get a motel room at night. You know? Trying to get enough money to eat because you spent it all.

Despite having known Barbara for several years at that point, this was the first time I had heard this story, reflecting the deep stigma associated with addictions.

Among other families, moving into the shelter seemed to be one stop in a cycle of mobility conditioned by a constellation of low-wage work, lack of affordable housing, and fragile relationships (see chapter 3). Nancy described the months leading up to her stay at Safe Harbor:

I was pregnant with [my son]. And his father—my ex-husband—and I were just dating at the time, and we broke up, and his brother and sister-in-law—we were living with them—they kicked me out. And I ended up in the [shelter].

Abigail recounted similarly precarious relationships and living situations before coming to Safe Harbor. After giving birth to her daughter, she and her boyfriend split up because "being a dad scared him." Abigail and the baby were living with her mother at the time:

And then me and my mom started fighting over parenting. So I moved out from there. I went to my best friend's house. So I lived there for a while. From there, I went to my uncle's and then back to my mom's. So then it was getting lonely. So my sister was always partying. We always had friends over. So I started hanging out with my sister. And I was doing some bad stuff, and I got pregnant with my son. So I got pregnant with him. I was living at my uncle's again, and I moved in with my best friend again, and I lived there 'til a week before I had my son. And then I moved back to my mom's 'cause some of stuff from their family went on. And my mom just didn't like the kids being there, so she kicked me out with both kids. So from there, I applied to the shelter. And I had a meeting with [shelter staff], and she accepted me. So we moved in. . . . It's kinda stunk, kinda ruined my respect for my mom—kicking me out with two kids and nowhere to go. But it's made me realize you can't really count on people even if it's your family. Which sucks, but—you need better.

Most of the families that I worked with had extended kin in the area. This fact surprised me greatly in the early months of my fieldwork. Going into this work, I had imagined "homeless families" as occupying a space far outside of the bonds of kin and had expected to hear about experiences of extrusion and separation from extended family networks, similar to the experiences of Euro-American participants with serious mental illness in previous research (Carpenter-Song et al., 2010). As I encountered the reality of parents, grandparents, and siblings in the local area, I was confronted with my own orientations toward the meaning of *family*. Although I was well aware that not all family dynamics are salubrious (Carpenter-Song, 2009a; Garcia, 2008; Jenkins, 1988; Jenkins & Csordas, 2020), it still seemed unimaginable to me that parents and children were not being taken in by extended family and found themselves living in a shelter. Dictating into my audio-recorder after visiting with a family one evening early in the research, I found myself wondering, *How could a grandmother allow her grandkids to live in a shelter?* What I would come to see over time is that my early interpretations, in addition to leaning dangerously on the precipice of judgment, misapprehended the various forms of support—and, in some cases, harm—that extended families offered.

As I would come to learn, in the midst of a housing crisis, families commonly turned to kin, friends, and acquaintances for shelter. Yet extended kin often lacked the resources to house and provide basic necessities for these adult children and their families. As such, families did not expect to be taken in for prolonged periods and were matter-of-fact as they stated, "My parents don't have room for all of us," or "My family can't afford to have us there." There was no expectation of long-term support from kin. As Nancy explained, "With the two kids, I really can't live at home. I mean, my mom just got rid of two kids [Nancy's siblings]. She's got one left at home. I don't think she needs the three of us moving in." In a striking corrective to the ungenerous portrait I had initially painted in my mind of her extended family, however, throughout the study Nancy's mother maintained regular contact, provided rides to run errands or go to health appointments, and was frequently tapped for groceries or diapers when money ran short.

For others, the presence of extended family in the area created continued points of vulnerability. As she reflected on their troubled relationship, Barbara confided that when she was growing up, her mother told her that she "didn't feel an instant love" when Barbara was born. This childhood wound remained painful for Barbara, and she asked longingly, "What kind of person says that?" Barbara's mother was unsympathetic when the family lost their home and, despite her own financial comfort, was not willing to take the family in.

The families' experiences offer insight into the range of circumstances surrounding a housing crisis and homelessness. As these experiences make clear, there is no single path that leads a family into homelessness. Indeed, to speak of pathways overlays a sense of linearity onto experiences that are instead a thorny tangle—a gradual accretion of misfortune, the subtle erosion of relationships, or the incremental fraying of a life shadowed by trauma and mental illness. As Vissing (1996) has observed:

> Homelessness is not a singular event or merely the lack of housing . . . homelessness is a *process* in which personal chaos occurs slowly, incrementally. Chaos, then, is the spiral of losing job, money, support networks, material possessions, and self-esteem, which ultimately results in the catastrophe of homelessness. (pp. 3–4)

This more nuanced view is an invitation into the complexity of rural housing insecurity.

Rhythm of Life at the Shelter

Arriving at the shelter after dark in the winter, I always saw several cars in the parking lot sending out puffs of exhaust like breath into the chilled air. I came to recognize a rhythm as engines would run for several minutes, fall silent, and then be coaxed again into a low purr. This oscillation was a sign of occupancy: someone was living in that vehicle and was toggling between a few minutes of warmth and a restless sleep. As I passed such cars, I instinctively averted my gaze from the car windows, preserving what I hoped was a small measure of privacy for its occupant.

I came to know the Safe Harbor shelter through other rhythms—the pull of a smoke break bringing mothers outdoors to congregate at the picnic table; the arrival of shouts and swiftly moving bodies as kids poured out of the school bus, breaking the languid quiet of the afternoon; the steady flow of cars throughout the day as men and women, young and old, came to the food pantry on the first floor of the shelter. Many people were greeted by name, part a cast of familiar characters around the shelter. Others were obviously new to the process, their eyes anxious and searching, their relief palpable as one of the shelter volunteers invited them to sit for a brief set of questions—"How large is your family? Please mark your income"—before accompanying them down a short hallway to a set of rooms lined with shelves stocked with cans of vegetables, tubs of peanut butter, boxes of cereal and pasta, and bins of fresh fruit.

The khaki clapboard structure and grounds of Safe Harbor, with edible gardens tended by a steadfast corps of volunteers during the short northern growing season, lacked the institutional feel that one might expect of a homeless shelter. The building seamlessly blended into the mix of houses and small businesses that lined the street. Safe Harbor housed up to eight families at a time. *Guests* (the preferred organizational term for residents of the shelter) occupied the second floor of Safe Harbor, with the space divided into two mirror-image *pods* housing four families each. Access to the second floor was restricted to shelter staff, resident families, and a limited set of others, such as doctors giving health presentations. I fell into this category of approved others and was granted full access by the executive director to spend time with families in the pods.

Unlike many shelters where people must queue up for space on a daily basis, at Safe Harbor families typically stayed for months at a time. It was common for families to be in residence at the shelter for six to nine months while they searched for housing, a timeline that underscores the lack of affordable housing within the region. Demand for space within the shelter was high, and vacated rooms were almost immediately filled by another family. Each family had two adjoining rooms—one room with bunkbeds for the children and the second room with a full-size bed for the parent(s). The four families on each pod shared two bathrooms, a kitchen, a dining table, and a common area with couches. With the pods configured in this way, families moved between the private space of their room and the shared, common areas.

Unlike the restricted-access pods, the first floor of the shelter was remarkably open to the community. Aside from a volunteer at the desk who conducted intake surveys for the food pantry, there were no gatekeepers as one usually expects to find in an institutional or service setting, no plexiglass barriers, and no signs demanding ID. During the day, people came and went through the main areas of the shelter—grabbing a cup of coffee in the cafe, using the shower facilities, catching up with shelter staff, or using the computer to search for jobs or housing. There were usually a few people smoking in the gazebo or outside the front entrance.

The organizational ethos of Safe Harbor strived to be family-centered, which, early in the study, the executive director contrasted for me with a paternalistic approach. As this organizational orientation played out for families, day-to-day life was not typically experienced as governed by rules and institutional rigidity. This flexibility was generally appreciated by families, although problems arose from the lack of more explicit structures. Barbara, for example, complained bitterly about having to live with "slobs" who did not pick up after themselves. Other residents expressed similar frustrations and grew resentful when assigned chores went undone. Many wished that staff members would more strictly monitor and enforce the expectation that families would engage in daily chores to keep the common areas and bathrooms clean.

Overall, I found the ethos of the organization to be individualistic rather than collectivist, with the nucleated American family very much in evidence despite the communal setting. While anthropologists have raised important critiques about strict dichotomies between *individualistic* and *collectivist* orientations in terms of cross-cultural comparisons that may essentialize cultures (Strauss, 2000), my use of these terms here describes a set of organizational expectations and practices that reflect the prioritization of the individual parent or family rather than the broader social group or collective. Staff members described the approach within the shelter as being strongly oriented to the individual choices of the guests, as Beth, a case manager at the shelter, explained:

> Our job is to really give them a leg up—help them to help themselves—and move forward in terms of finding housing, getting a job, or going to school or whatever it may be. So we have a lot of programs that we use to help people move along. I mean, ultimately, it's the person's choice. . . . The key is that the guests have to want to improve themselves. I mean, it's their choice. Our whole system is based on choices. And the rules that we do have and guidelines that we do have are based on choices the guests make.

The individualistic orientation within the shelter was reflected in daily routines within the pods. Families generally prepared their own meals and ate in shifts rather than preparing a common meal together.[6] Networks of sharing—with food, cigarettes, babysitting—were formally discouraged by the shelter staff. Beyond discouraging the sharing of material resources, I heard stories from several participants about how shelter staff members had discouraged them from "counseling" each other. From the guests' perspectives, this limited significant sources of support from those with similar life experiences:

> Me and [fellow guest] had quite a conversation a couple of nights ago. I was very, very upset, and [staff member], of course, told me that it wasn't right for me to talk to [guest]. That she is not my counselor—that I shouldn't be doing things like that. And I just felt, like—I just felt, like, you know, these are my friends. I consider them my family. My dorm family. And outside of this place, I hope that if we ever do live apart, then I'd like to keep in touch. But to sit there and say that what is my personal thoughts and my personal opinions—she has no right to say that I can't speak to who I wanna speak to. I mean, if I wanted to go see a counselor, I'd go see a counselor. But it won't make me feel better because they're just there to listen. With a friend, it's *comfort*. And she [staff member] doesn't see it that way. She sees it as, "Oh, this is someone that lives with you, and they don't have to know your business."

Despite such criticisms, guests were generally deeply appreciative of living at Safe Harbor and found it to be a supportive environment, as Melissa, a young mother, described:

> My kids are happy. They like it here, and *I* like it here. And besides the fact that I'm homeless, it's very positive. There's a lot of positive energy. There's always someone for you to talk to. They always have different things that you can do. [They] work

with you on this, work with you on that. And—just the support. There's lots and lots of support, and I don't—where I'm from, I didn't have any of that.

Kate, another guest, shared her perspectives on the shelter environment:

I mean, I like the support. I like the groups that they have down on Wednesdays and Fridays. It's a lot of fun. I mean, they help you with the food shelf, and if you need something in a pinch, they'll help you with that.

As Melissa and Kate's comments highlight, "support" within the shelter setting entailed access to material resources, the efforts of staff to "work with" shelter guests, and the sense of "positive energy" within the organization, activities, and groups.

Echoing the individualistic orientation of the shelter more broadly, housing searches were all done by each individual family rather than through a more collectivist approach that would allow families to combine income and share costs after leaving the shelter. This strategy may reflect state and federal housing subsidy regulations and local ordinances but also underscores unquestioned cultural orientations that privilege the primacy of the nuclear family in the United States. In practical terms, this may represent a significant missed opportunity to facilitate the pooling of resources, especially in a local context marked by high rents and limited housing inventory.

Against the backdrop of few affordable housing options, families at the shelter spent a great deal of time filling out housing applications. They recognized that most of this effort was futile but were propelled by the hope of "getting a break" as well as the requirements of the shelter that they maintain an active search for housing, as one guest described:

They want you to do a certain amount: like, 20 hours a week they want you to look. Sometimes you look in the paper, and it's, like, you can't *afford* these places, and they still want you to write 'em down so they know that you're looking.

Staff members assisted guests with housing paperwork and with potential leads through word-of-mouth connections to landlords and local housing authorities. Guests also emphasized that the housing search required a great deal of personal effort: "You've gotta do a lot on your own." I understood such narratives of personal effort and tenacity as expressions of moral worthiness (Snell-Rood & Carpenter-Song, 2018) as they often existed alongside comparisons to others at the shelter, who were criticized for "wanting everything handed to them." On our way to run errands together, Tara would take the opportunity to place follow-up calls to landlords. "You've gotta be persistent," she explained. She had been waiting for months for one land-lord to approve her application for a two-bedroom apartment: "I've done everything that *I* need to do. Now it's just waiting on paperwork and stuff." She struggled to remain hopeful in the face of interminable bureaucratic delays to be approved for a subsidized housing complex.

For parents with young children, the rhythm of the days at the shelter was a slow one that was oriented toward the intimate tasks of caring for babies and toddlers. Parents often commented on how "boring" it was and how "there's nothing to do." During the days, the atmosphere was quiet. Most families spent time in their rooms rather than in the common living areas. Afternoons were often spent watching videos with their small children and dozing together. When families gathered together in the common areas in the hours after school and around dinnertime, the small children tended to make their own fun. For school-age children, their days were organized around going to school and attending the shelter's after-school program, where they finished their homework, read, and played games.

One day early in my fieldwork, I was visiting with Nancy and Abigail and their toddler-age daughters. The midafternoon sun slanted through the windows of the common room as yawns went around the kitchen table like dominoes. Nancy greeted me with a warm, "Hey, Elizabeth," and Abigail smiled as I joined them at the table. She nodded in the direction of the high chair, "You can meet Mary." The little girl, 19 months old, was sitting in front of a plate of rice and bananas. "Oh, look at that hair!" I said, admiring the girl's two tiny pigtails. I reached into my bag for the snacks that I had brought for the children—Goldfish crackers and animal cookies in circus train boxes. Nancy immediately noticed, "Oh look, Emily! She brought your favorite!" As little Emily climbed up on my lap, I joked, "I know the way to this one's heart." Nancy conferred, "Yeah, if you've got food, you're gonna be her best friend." I opened the box and placed three cookies on the table, which Emily snatched in her dimpled hand before sliding down from her chair. As always, Emily was up and down and up and down. When a staff member, Anne, came into the pod, Emily rushed over to her. Anne danced with her—a modified "quick step," she would later joke—and Emily mimicked her movements, toddling back and forth.

I was constantly aware of the presence of others at the shelter. When I arrived one evening with a pizza to share with Jim and his four young children, I was soon confronted with the awkwardness of other families in the common dining area as I brought in dinner. A woman quickly ushered her young son away—"That's not for you"—as he looked on longingly. This was so different from my previous work with families in which the privacy of the family home was a given. Unlike this earlier work, in which conversations could stretch long into the evening and delve into the personal and deeply sensitive, when I was with families at the shelter, our interactions largely consisted of small talk and the stuff of daily routines. Without ever making this explicit, we found other ways and other spaces to share more intimate and often painful experiences. My car became such a space. Rather than hanging out at the shelter, parents would often ask me to take them to run errands or would suggest that we go out for coffee. Especially for those with limited means of transportation, this was a welcome opportunity to leave the shelter.

The presence of other families and staff members in daily life underscores that families experiencing homelessness give up the autonomy and privacy of American family life. As Donna Friedman (2000) aptly describes it, homeless families must "parent in public." For families at the shelter, the basic activities of everyday life—eating, bathing, sleeping—became subject to monitoring through the eyes of shelter staff. Shelter staff described feeling conflicted when they observed parenting practices that differed from their own experiences, and some offered thoughtful reflections on their discomfort that acknowledged not wanting to impose "middle-class standards" on families living in poverty. Our anthropological training prepares us to suspend our own cultural orientations, and, as a psychological anthropologist, I was familiar with the vast range of child-rearing practices around the world. Yet I shared this sense of discomfort when I witnessed harsh words spoken to a small child or conversations veering toward sex or drinking within earshot of young children, and I actively reflected in order to bracket my own experiences and assumptions.

"Parenting in public" (Friedman, 2000) also meant that families' lives were subject to the judgments of fellow residents of the shelter. Barbara criticized some of the young mothers at Safe Harbor who, in her view, did not engage and interact with their children enough:

> You've got all that time, you know. I would take my kids when they were little, put 'em in the stroller, go for a walk, just—you know, *do things*. You read, you play, you know? You play with them. [The mothers at the shelter] don't have any desire like that. . . .

From her perspective, this was evidence of selfishness, as she continued:

> And these young mothers today, that's what it is—all about them. Has nothing to
> do with those poor children they bring into this world. And that's what I see. It's
> "poor me, poor this and that." . . . Their lives are not about taking care of those
> children. It's about everything else that's going on in the world. And this kid just
> came along and ruined my fun. And it's sad because that's your next generation.

Reflecting on a similar set of observations, Jim and Hannah offered a more
generous interpretation:

Jim: I saw very few parents that *played* with their kids. I mean, just 'cause
their heads were just so *consumed* by everything that was going on.

Hannah: The drama in their relationships.

Jim: Yeah, *drama* is one thing and then just the—the stressors of being homeless, and they lose that peace.

Drama was a word commonly invoked to describe the interpersonal rhythms
of families at the shelter. For many, life appeared to be lived in sharp contrast, with families oscillating between highs and lows. The emotional lives
of families tended to ebb and flow between hope, relief, and celebration, on
one hand, and disappointment, worry, and despair, on the other.

Social Responses to Vulnerability

The urgency of moralistic discourses of good parenting must be understood
against the backdrop of the feelings of shame and impotence wrought by
homelessness. Driving back to the shelter after running errands one evening, Tara described her relief at finally being on the brink of moving into
her own apartment:

Tara: So I won't be at Safe Harbor anymore. . . . I won't be a homeless person anymore. I'm definitely happy. This chick that works at [restaurant] I
used to be friends with her, and I guess she went and told somebody, "Oh,
I try not to talk to her and [Tara's husband] anymore since they've been
homeless."

ECS: Really?

Tara: Holy shit, what a bitch. Yeah, . . . it pissed me off. I'd like to smash
her face. (sighs) Really irritated. . . . People are like that—treat you like shit
'cause you live in a homeless shelter. It's not even that I'm homeless. It's 'cause
I live in a homeless shelter, and it makes me a bad person. I don't know,

but whatever. She worked at the [restaurant]. Her name's [deleted]. She's a dumb bitch. If you ever have her as a waitress, don't tip her.

In Tara's narrative, we hear her actively working through the nuanced categorical distinctions of homelessness, navigating a terrain dense with social rejection, shame, and resistance. She begins by noting an imminent shift away from being a "homeless person" as she anticipates leaving Safe Harbor. A few sentences later, she makes a subtle distinction between being "homeless" and "living in a homeless shelter." This distinction, though perhaps not fully intentional or conscious, creates a space for the disentanglement of "homeless" as something attached to one's identity. Instead, "living in a homeless shelter" is a circumstance. While it would seem that viewing homelessness as a (temporary) set of circumstances instead of a (fixed) identity would mitigate social rejection and stigma, Tara's narrative clearly upends such assumptions.

In the rural New England context in which self-sufficiency and hard work are core values, those who become homeless may be viewed by those in their social networks as "failures" or "trash." Participants described painful rejections from former friends. Hannah's voice was tinged with bitterness as she recounted how her friends "evaporated" when "the shit hit the fan," despite this being the time when she "needed a friend the most": "And they realized that I was really serious and I had a really serious problem. Then they all ran scared, and once that was gone, there was absolutely—I had no outlet. I had nothing!" As Hannah and her family faced eviction, "They wouldn't let their kids play with my kids. One girl's husband wouldn't let her talk to me anymore. They stopped answering their phones."

The sting of such rejection may be exacerbated by the lack of anonymity in rural settings. In small towns, vulnerabilities are likely to be known by those around you. Families in the study tried hard to maintain privacy regarding hardships they were experiencing. Barbara never told her own mother that she and her children stayed in a shelter for nine months, saying simply, "I'm too ashamed." She enjoyed our time together because she did not have to conceal this information:

> it's been so nice and refreshing to come out and *talk* with somebody. Because my own, my own friends and things like that, you know—homeless is not something you truly want to admit to being, you know? Nobody at my work knows that, or anything, you know? But it's been *very* refreshing to come out and be able to talk to somebody, you know to just to . . . let it out. . . .

Some families chose to cut off ties to others and avoided social situations to steel themselves against the effects of pernicious gossip and embarrassment. Public interactions were inevitably fraught for these families as running into acquaintances or engaging in innocuous small talk risked exposing the reality of their plight. When Jim and Hannah attended a chili cook-off in their community, they found that they had difficulty meeting and talking to people. Hannah explained, "I have trouble with that now. I didn't use to have trouble with that." Jim elaborated how he cannot have a "normal" conversation with anyone: "If you start to tell people about it, they back off because they have preconceptions: we must've just gotten kicked out of our trailer park." Jim's narrative draws attention to the reservoir of stigmatizing associations with poverty and housing insecurity among others in the Upper Valley community and the expectation of rejection if the reality of their situation was exposed.

Yet it was also the case that Jim would occasionally distance himself from those in similarly precarious circumstances. He was an avid reader. Milk crates filled to the brim with books were precious cargo that accompanied their many moves. As we sat together in a motel room after the family had left Safe Harbor, he commented, "I don't know how I'd deal with our situation if I wasn't educated." At times, other participants rendered harsh judgments of others at Safe Harbor. Tara spoke derisively of "those people" at the shelter as "losers and takers." Similarly, Barbara compared herself to others at the shelter who "sit around" and "sleep all day." Such moralizing discourses simultaneously reinforced stereotypes of people living in poverty and also served as a means of asserting their own moral worth (cf. Snell-Rood & Carpenter-Song, 2018).

Beyond the responses of friends and associates and the broader public reactions to homelessness, it is worthwhile to examine the complex and often mixed responses to extreme financial precarity among extended kin. At the beginning of this chapter, I called attention to the forms of help and harm manifest in extended family relations. Throughout the study, Nancy frequently appealed to her mother to buy groceries and toiletries. These requests often came at the end of the month when money—and food—typically ran short. In some instances, such requests were met with warmth, as Nancy described an afternoon spent together: "My mom was really nice to me the other day. 'Cause she ended up buying me a pack of cigarettes, took us out to lunch. I was like, 'Holy cow.'" As Nancy's surprise suggests, requests for help were not always fulfilled, and family members could be capricious in their responses. One afternoon, after her mother had refused such an appeal, Nancy was frustrated: "I was only asking for one thing for myself, and that was toilet paper. Everything else was for the kids [diapers] and the cats [cat food]."

In Nancy's case, later in the study her extended family provided substantial financial assistance. Her grandparents contributed the money for a security deposit on an apartment as an "investment" in the young family: "They're so happy for us. They brought cookies over for us [in the new apartment]." Months later, as Nancy's marriage dissolved, and she faced eviction, her parents paid her rent. As the months wore on, her parents' patience wore thin, and Nancy resented feeling like a burden: "I told my mom: 'Don't get mad at me. I am doing everything that I can to keep my head above water. If you want to get mad at somebody, get mad at the deadbeat who left me.'" Yet it was clearly not sustainable for her parents to continue paying her market-rate rent of $800 per month. At other times, Nancy voiced awareness of the strain these forms of financial support put on her parents: "I hate asking my mom for money to help me out because, you know, these [diapers] aren't cheap. I think that these are about $20, . . . and she also bought a can of formula for, like, $27." One evening, as tears streamed down her cheeks, Nancy said simply: "I should be able to do this on my own. I shouldn't need to ask my mom for help."

Family Portrait: Subjective Experience and Personal Meanings of Homelessness

Amid cultural values and expectations of self-reliance, the profound social stigma faced by families experiencing homelessness was recast as shame and personal failure in parents' subjective experience. Families surviving in poverty in rural New England are largely alienated from the signifiers of "the good life" in the United States—a nice house, a steady income, stable relationships, reliable transportation. Not having a stable home was experienced by many families as a personal failure that struck at the core of what it means to be a good parent.

One evening, I sat with Jim and Hannah, a married couple in their 40s with four children, and I asked them to share their perspectives on the experience and meaning of being a mother and a father. The question became a point of departure for them to open up to me about the specific impacts of homelessness as a parent. Hannah spoke to the tensions between their focus on day-to-day survival and the need to support her children. She expressed her own sense of deep vulnerability and fear of failing her children:

Hannah: Well, I think the biggest challenge is that when you face homelessness [long pause] as a parent— . . . your focus has to be so much on, like, surviving, that it's so easy to lose sight of what really, really needs to be done. And, and you were talking about being a, a father, being a mother. I mean, that was my biggest—and that's been my biggest struggle. How do I survive, and how do I be a mother, how do I support my kids? I feel so completely vulnerable. . . . I think I still really struggle with my tendencies to totally withdraw away from my children out of complete fear that I'm gonna completely fail.

At this point, Jim entered the dialogue, and the couple elaborated on their subjective sense of failure. In the rush of their words, the high stakes of parenting in poverty became palpable as they articulated the gap between the fierce desire to protect and shelter their children and the cruel reality of housing insecurity:

Jim: Well, you feel like you have failed. Once you reach that point of not having—

Hannah [overlapping]: Oh, yeah! You completely fail! I mean, it's, it's, "What have I done?" You know?

Jim: The biggest drive is to protect your children and make sure that they're, they're, they're sheltered.

Hannah: Right. Yeah. Appropriate shelter, which is not a shelter. . . . It's not a hotel room.

In her words, Hannah draws a distinction between physical shelter—a homeless shelter or a hotel room—and what she terms "appropriate" shelter. Over the years that I knew them, Jim and Hannah aspired to provide "appropriate" shelter—a home of their own—for their children.[7] Building on their descriptions of the subjective sense of failure, Jim spoke to the emotional and psychological toll of not being able to "fix what's wrong":

Jim: 'Cause I think once you hit that point [of losing your home], you really feel very stuck. 'Cause you can't just fix it. And when you're looking at your kids, and you can't fix what's wrong, it's, . . . you know—it's, it's, it's automatically just gonna create all kinds of emotional, psychological, just baggage.

As the light outside faded to darkness, the conversation turned to how homelessness had impacted their young children. For Jim and Hannah's children, losing their home upended their relationships and ties within the community. I was struck by the foreclosing of opportunities to engage in the quotidian activities of childhood as a hidden consequence of deep poverty and homelessness:

Hannah: I mean, my children are coming to me—my daughter was coming to me with, "How?" You know? "Why, Mommy?" You know? I mean, she can't have her little friends come over to play. You know, she can't invite one of her girlfriends to spend the night. I mean, she can't—

Jim: Can't take them out to the movie, you can't—

Hannah: She can't talk to—yeah, we can't go to movies, we can't go to the park, we can't go skating, we can't go bowling, we can't—you know. And then, because she doesn't wanna, she didn't wanna meet anybody and be not normal. And then, I feel the same way! I lost my friends! So how am I supposed to explain that to them? I mean, you know? I found myself sitting in a chair yesterday with my daughter just in tears. And she cried for an hour, and I'm in tears with her! I did not know what to say to her. You know? I couldn't tell her that it's gonna be okay because I didn't know if it's gonna be okay.

Their account—with its steady chorus of "can't"—illuminates the cascade of losses that accompanies financial devastation and homelessness for families. Hannah's account underscores the shared familial experience of loss ("I feel the same way! I lost my friends!") and also how homelessness may erode the desire to participate and interact with others for fear of not being "normal." Her daughter's fear of meeting other people echoes Jim and Hannah's earlier descriptions of not being able to have a "normal conversation" with anyone in the community because of the expectation of stigma and social rejection.

Jim and Hannah described their subjective experience of homelessness as a process of withdrawal. Over time, the layering of losses appears to gradually extinguish motivation:

Jim: You very much withdraw with the whole threat of homelessness. And once you're there, you do withdraw. You don't interact, and your situation just—

Hannah [interjecting]: You don't wanna go back to school, you don't wanna look for a job. You don't pay bills because even opening up the bills is so stressful.

Jim: Oh yeah, money's a huge thing. . . . You have so little you really cease to care. Um, 'cause you've been without and completely without. . . . But you look at it, and you think, "Well this might be gone tomorrow. What difference does it make?"

For this couple, material losses and financial precarity catalyzed shifts in subjective experience away from engagement and participation toward withdrawal and apathy. Yet Jim and Hannah did not fully succumb to the forces of withdrawal. Rather, they continued in their daily efforts to meet their family's basic survival needs. Their ongoing efforts underscore the role of "struggle" (Jenkins, 2015b; Jenkins & Csordas, 2020) in the midst of suffering. Struggle, in this sense, "goes beyond the useful and increasingly prominent notion of individual resilience in the face of affliction" (Jenkins, 2015a, p. 2) by instead viewing "the human capacity for struggle as a fundamental human process of vigorously engaging possibility" (Jenkins & Csordas, 2020, p. 7).

Building on these insights, Jim and Hannah's experience also reveals a possible shadow side to struggle that is manifest in the emotional and bodily fallout of housing insecurity. They described their utter exhaustion as they worked to patch together resources for survival and days consumed by efforts to meet their family's basic needs:

Jim: Then you gotta go—somebody wants to meet with you before they agree they're gonna help you with something. So then you gotta drive to wherever they are. . . . You become consumed in just *surviving*, and as a parent it diminishes your ability to take care of your kids.

Hannah: I mean for five bucks! I mean stressing over *five dollars*.

Jim: And then at the end of the day, you're emotionally and sometimes physically *exhausted*. You're just wiped! I was going to bed at the same time my kids were 'cause I just didn't have the *oomph*.

Homelessness in Rural New England

To become homeless threatens the bodily and existential survival of families. The basics necessary to sustain life can no longer be taken for granted as efforts to secure food, clothing, and shelter occupy the principal daily energies of families experiencing homelessness. These families survive in the cast-off spaces at the margins of small New England towns. These rural "zones of abandonment," to borrow from João Biehl (2005), are the shabby motels, the remote, ramshackle houses, the cars, and the couches that families occupy as they struggle, scratch, and search for a semblance of security.

Families experiencing homelessness faced marginalization across settings and interactions in their everyday lives. Drawing on her ethnographic research among homeless women with serious mental illness in Chicago, anthropologist Tanya Luhrmann observes, "one thing is obvious, and that is that to be homeless—whether or not you are psychotic—is to confront social defeat daily and on many dimensions" (Luhrmann, 2007, p. 154). Social defeat occurs when individuals have consistent and repeated social interactions in which they experience failure—for example, "an encounter with another person who demeans them, humiliates them, subordinates them" (Luhrmann, 2007, p. 151). Families' experiences resonate with the "constant grind of humiliation, repudiation, and rejection" experienced by the homeless women in Luhrmann's (2007, p. 162) research. Researchers have found that homeless mothers, in particular, are vulnerable to being stigmatized as inadequate parents (Barrow & Laborde, 2008; Cosgrove & Flynn, 2005), and homeless women with children have been described as "the most demoralized of all adult homeless subgroups" (Buckner et al., 1993, p. 396). Yet it is also important to recognize that processes of social exclusion are not uniform across sociocultural settings, as Jocelyn Marrow and Tanya Luhrmann (2012) note:

> We believe that the zones of social abandonment that we find empirically—the social forms which anthropologists name and identify in the local worlds they study—bear the marks of their specific social location, and that when a community withdraws from those it abandons, it does so in socially specific ways. (p. 494)

In urban settings, such social defeat occurs largely in anonymous encounters— recalling Kim Hopper's observation that the "city's forsaken" are "each studiously ignored by passersby" (2003, p. 3). By contrast, the lack of anonymity in small-town New England means that experiences of social defeat are often catalyzed by those who know you. In turn, homelessness brings immense shame as families confront snubs, insults, and humiliations in their everyday encounters with friends, neighbors, and family members.

The aftermath of a housing crisis was fraught with rejection, isolation, and shame. Becoming homeless in this setting means not only the loss of home but also, for many, the eventual and seemingly inevitable dissolution of social ties and deep strains on relationships. Families were discarded by friends in subtle ways, manifesting in unanswered phones, insulting comments, and refusals to help in times of need. Family members offered help when they could but faced limits on their own finances and patience in the context of continued need. Looking broadly at the Upper Valley, outpourings of support are common, with community members rallying around families that have suffered a tragic death, a house fire, or other such public tragedy. But for families that exhibit chronic need, there seems to be a limit to sympathy for those who cannot make it on their own. Moreover, those living in poverty largely ascribe to cultural expectations that they *should* be able to make it on their own.

Following from this, characteristics of the rural New England cultural context shape families' experiences of social exclusion and families' responses to homelessness and poverty. Self-reliance is a deeply engrained cultural orientation in the United States that shapes experiences of vulnerability and expectations for recovery (Myers, 2015), and this sensibility is especially pronounced in rural New England. By contrast, studies of poverty and housing insecurity in Appalachia have found a strong emphasis on family ties and a "take-care-of-our-own" philosophy (Shamblin et al., 2012, p. 5). Those who experience a housing crisis in Appalachia are typically welcomed in by kin (Shamblin et al., 2012). Similarly, Elizabeth Lindsey (1996) found that families in nonmetropolitan Georgia received assistance from their family and friends in the process of restabilization following homelessness. In their research examining how families reintegrate following homelessness, Katherine Dunlap and Sondra Fogel (1998) noted the importance of a caring community to support families following an episode of homelessness.

The prevailing ethos of individualism and self-sufficiency in this New England setting (cf. Markus & Conner, 2013) holds implications for how individuals understand and respond to adversity, what their expectations are for receiving help, to whom it is appropriate to turn in times of need, and how long this help should be available. The families with whom I have worked were not embraced by the proverbial village during times of need. Support from kin was generous at times but unreliable as family members faced their own financial difficulties or grew frustrated when adult children could not make it on their own. In this setting, the loss of housing is frequently cast as a personal failure within one's social network and is also, tragically, a view often internalized by the displaced themselves. Parents ascribed to expectations of self-reliance amid structural forces that seriously constrained their ability to make it on their own. I describe this cultural orientation as the *New England bootstrap mentality* in reference to the paradigmatic—and deeply problematic—expression of individualism and self-sufficiency.[8] Throughout the remaining chapters, I endeavor to illuminate how the bootstrap mentality informs families' experiences of poverty and housing insecurity as well as their engagements with institutions of care.

3   Life on the Edge

By March 2010, all five of the families in the study had exited the shelter. All had been guests at Safe Harbor for between six to nine months, a typical length of stay at the shelter. Housing arrangements and circumstances of leaving the shelter varied among the families: Abigail, Tara, and Barbara all moved with their families directly into subsidized apartments; Nancy reunited with her former boyfriend, and they moved into a rented townhome with another couple; Jim and Hannah, following the removal of their children by the Department of Children and Families, no longer qualified for a room at the family shelter and initially moved into a local motel and then, three months later, into a Section 8 rental home. While I did not recognize it at the time, these various settings—subsidized and market-rate housing, pay-by-the-week motels, and informal doubling up—would appear over and over again in the course of the study. In thinking back to the spring of 2010, I remember being buoyed by the optimism of many of the families as they anticipated fresh starts. Particularly for the families moving into subsidized housing, this seemed to be a story of success—the confluence of a supportive service environment, the good fortune of affordable housing availability, and patience and persistence on the part of the families.

In the spring of 2010. I was also approaching the horizon of the original timeline for the project, which had been designed initially as a short-term exploratory study of rural homelessness. With all of the families now housed, a question arose: was I still studying homelessness? This was the beginning of the blurred edges that would continue to characterize this research. Most studies of family homelessness concentrate on the periods of time when families meet federal definitions of homelessness or when they are in shelters (Friedman, 2000; Kozol, 2011). The boundedness of this work on family homelessness contrasts with studies of rural poverty and housing insecurity that emphasize the fluidity of families' experiences across housing settings (Fitchen, 1992; Vissing, 1996). Propelled in part by the knowledge of the spurious distinction between those who are poor and those who become homeless in rural areas (Fitchen, 1992; Whitley, 2013) but in greater measure by a desire to maintain connections with people whom I had grown to know and to care about and who had invited me into their lives and vulnerabilities, I made the decision to continue the work of documenting families' experiences in the community following their initial episode of homelessness.

As I witnessed and participated in the lives of families over time, I became aware of oscillating rhythms of stability and instability. The swell of optimism and hope I felt in the spring of 2010 receded as families endured persistent threats to their housing security, struggled to get by on service-sector wages, and faced isolation and stigma in rural communities. For these families, their lives were suffused by what I describe as *fundamental insecurity*. This concept strives to evoke the totality and pervasiveness of instability, impermanence, and mobility in the lives of families that have experienced homelessness. As such, this concept is positioned as an inverse of what Deborah Padgett (2007, p. 1926) has described as the "ontological security" that formerly homeless people experience when they have a home, manifested in a sense of control, constancy, reassuring daily routines, privacy, and conditions that support identity construction and repair. In this chapter, I examine how fundamental insecurity manifests in conditions of chronic housing insecurity, precarious forms of work, profound financial scarcity, and fragile relationships. I also explore how families continue to endure and cultivate meaning in their lives in the context of precarity. In doing so, I apply anthropological theories of "moral striving" (Mattingly, 2014) and "struggle" (Jenkins, 2015b; Jenkins & Csordas, 2020) to illuminate efforts to cultivate stability for their families amid the long shadows of fundamental insecurity.

Family Portraits of Mobility

Abigail

"I'm moving out!" Abigail's excitement was palpable in the spring of 2010 as she told me that she and her children would soon be moving out of Safe Harbor into a subsidized apartment about 20 miles south. Abigail was 19 at the time, White, and raising her daughter, Mary, who was just shy of two-years-old and her son, Adam, who had been born a few months earlier. She was a single mother and maintained contact with her children's fathers. The sun streamed through the windows of the common room as we chatted. "It's beautiful," she said, her round face breaking into a wide smile. "It used to be really bad down there [at the apartment complex], but they gutted the place last year." Abigail and her kids had been at Safe Harbor for five months.

The next time we saw each other, Abigail had moved out of the shelter, and she welcomed me into her new apartment. She looked rested and fresh-faced with her long hair pulled back into a ponytail, accentuating her youth. Dressed in leggings and new sneakers, she embodied a sense of a fresh start. "It's very quiet. I met a couple of the neighbors. They're really nice." The unit smelled of fresh paint and new carpet as Abigail gave me a brief tour. "Wow, this is a big space," I commented. "So you've got two bedrooms?" She corrected me, "Three. Yeah, so we put the kids together, and then they have a little toy room, too." Since moving into the apartment, Abigail had noticed changes with her son: "Since we moved, he's been eating so much better. Like, his naps are so much better. And his sleeping—like, he sleeps in his crib." I asked her what she thinks the difference was, and she reflected, "I think it's just more calm here. Like, I'm not stressed. It can get a bit lonely, but, I mean, I read a lot, which is nice. 'Cause at the shelter, I'd wanna go hang out with someone. But I think now I'm not stressed or worried about meetings or stuff."

This marked the first time that Abigail had lived on her own with Mary and Adam. Prior to Safe Harbor, Abigail had moved back and forth between her mother's and sister's houses, where she had experienced a mix of support and strain (see chapter 2). While she welcomed the calm environment at the new apartment, she also found it challenging to live far from her family and friends:

Abigail: It's different. I mean, I don't really see my family, so . . . [trails off].

ECS: Has that been tough?

Abigail: Um, kinda, 'cause my mom's been really sick. She's been in the hospital. [pause] But it's okay. Other than that, my sisters have been down, and my friend's family comes down to see me. And then my uncle and my aunt come over for dinner, so—[pause] It's different. Coming in *my* house for dinner. And then I have to cook! And I'm like, "Oh God!"

[both laugh]

ECS: What are you gonna make?

Abigail: We're having cheeseburgers and salad. So it'll be fun. [My son] gets to see his little cousins. . . . Other than that, I don't really have anyone down here. Don't really know anyone. Don't really go anywhere. But it's nice, though. I like having my own little house. And cleaning and stuff.

ECS: Is this the first time you've had a place of your own?

Abigail: Yeah. I mean, I love my family and friends, but this is *my* place now.

ECS: So what's that like for you? That's a big transition.

Abigail: Yeah, it's so weird. Like, I dunno. At the shelter, I was used to every morning waking up, and, you know, someone will be around, and I had coffee with someone. And now I wake up to—it's just [my kids]. But it's nice, though. There's no screaming, there's no fighting. A couple of neighbors that I've talked to, they come down, and they check on me. 'Cause I'm the youngest person here. [laughs] It's different. It's nice doing stuff. Not having to have rules and freaking out over, like, when are you gonna be home? It doesn't matter. It's so weird! Like, I don't do much. I just hang out, and my kids play, and I clean and . . . [trails off]. But I finally made it to my own place, which is *so* nice.

As the weeks went on, I noticed that Abigail spoke more and more about being lonely. The pride of having her own place was increasingly tempered by the isolation of spending most of her time alone in the apartment, tending to her small children. Despite the "drama" that had often ensued with others at Safe Harbor, she looked back fondly on many of her interactions with others at the shelter:

> Another good person [at the shelter] was Barbara. Like, at first I didn't really like her. [laughs] But I was smoking a cigarette one day, and we were really talking, and she had a lot of really good outlooks on life. Like, she helped me a lot when [my son] was sick and stuff, so. And she just helped me keep my head up, and you know, would remind me that, "No one's perfect."
>
> [The women's support] group was fun. . . . It was so nice just to have someone to talk to and just sit there and do crafts or talk or whatever. And there'd be daycare, so, like, you're kid-free, and so it was nice. And the staff didn't make you feel like—say, I go down to the clothing or food room, 'cause you needed a can of whatever. They [the staff] didn't make you feel bad for asking [for food or clothes]. . . . Like, they were just really nice about it if you ever needed anything. They'd help you. . . . They're just really respectful there, which is weird because a lot of places like that, they'll be, like, make you feel like you're, not worthy of it. I dunno, it was nice. I made a lot of good friends there.

A few months later, toward the end of the summer in 2010, Abigail and the kids moved out of the subsidized apartment. When I asked her about this decision, she said simply: "I just don't want to be by myself." The loneliness and boredom of being on her own had grown intolerable. Abigail and the kids moved into a house owned by her best friend's parents. The small, run-down house was located on a dirt road in a small Vermont town far from the main centers for employment, shopping, and healthcare in the region. In exchange for a shared room and access to transportation (driving Abigail to appointments or to run errands), Abigail paid them $140 in rent, a quarter of the utilities, and the entirety of her Supplemental Nutrition Assistance Program (SNAP) benefits for the household. Doubling up with her friend's family initially gave Abigail the support and company that she had craved. Her friend's mother took an active role in helping Abigail with childcare—feeding, changing diapers, and occasionally babysitting so that Abigail and her friend could enjoy an evening out at the Upper Valley's only night club.

But over time, the arrangement appeared to fall out of balance, and Abigail felt taken advantage of by her friend's parents. A month after moving in, she learned that the money she was paying in rent was going toward a vacation for her friend's family—not toward paying down the mortgage, which they were behind on. They had also used the bulk of Abigail's SNAP benefits to pay for food for the trip. Abigail felt torn: she wanted to move out but did not want to be alone again. The environment grew increasingly tense, and eventually Abigail felt uncomfortable staying any longer.

In November 2010, she and the kids moved in with another friend, a young mother of four. This arrangement lasted only a few weeks, ending when the friend's boyfriend became aggressive toward Abigail's children. In addition to losing housing, Abigail lost most of her clothes, her iPod, and a portable DVD player: "It was, like, all of my expensive stuff. And [my friend] was, like, 'Well, I'm keeping it.' And the cops won't do anything."

With the support of her welfare case manager, Abigail and the kids were placed in a motel. The two-story, 34-unit structure was built in the 1950s and served traveling salesmen and families passing through the railroad town of White River Junction, Vermont. In the ensuing decades, the motel transformed from a modest, AAA-rated establishment to a place better known for the frequency of its police activity (Hongoltz-Hetling, 2017) and dubbed "Heroin Hotel" (Kenyon, 2017). Abigail described the state of the room when she and the kids moved in:

> It is nasty. I have never lived in a nasty place. I would rather live at the shelter, okay? That is what I told the maintenance guy who changed my locks. Because, I said, "Can I have, like, new locks?" That was because I had no key. *They gave me no key.* When I got my room, there were beer bottles everywhere. There was stuff all over the bathroom.

With the help of a friend, Abigail cleaned the room and set about trying to settle in. She described the maintenance man's kindness in her early days at the motel, orienting her to the other people staying there and offering advice:

> He was really nice. He was, like, "Don't talk to this person. Don't talk to them. . . . They are good people, they have kids, you know?" . . . He was, like, "If you need anything, you can come and see me." And he was, like, "You are one of those responsible moms that gets stuck in a shitty situation." And I was, like, "Yeah, that tends to happen to me, or I make the wrong choices or whatever." But he is, like, "You know what? Your kids are with you. You have full custody." He was, like, "You are doing something." He told me to put up pictures for the kids. It makes them feel like you are comfortable here. So he told me to decorate. . . . He told me, "Just be sure you always have your kids with you. The DCYF [Department of Children, Youth, and Families] people come here all of the time."

As we sat together in the dingy room, Abigail took a long drag on her cigarette and sighed: "You've met with me in so many different places over the last year, Elizabeth."

Over the course of the winter, Abigail hoped to get back into Safe Harbor, where she would receive more support in finding housing:

> I called the [shelter]. And I'm trying to get back in there as much as I don't want to. But it is better than being here. . . . They set up, like, ten searches a week for apartments. I don't want to stay here [at the motel]. I really don't want to be homeless.

At the time, it was costing $280 per week to stay at the motel—a sum that she knew was exorbitant given the condition of the property. Yet she faced a catch-22 common to others in the study. Lacking the ability to pay a lump sum for a security deposit and for the first and last months' rent, she was trapped in a cycle of overpaying for substandard housing on a week-to-week basis.

By February 2011, Abigail had managed to save some money and was hoping to move out of the motel. Her plans and hopes were dashed when a boyfriend whom she had been dating for a few weeks stole her savings:

He was the first guy I have dated since I had [my son]. And I got fucked up so bad—all of my money and everything else. The money was my main thing. It took a lot of time to save that up. And he knew how much I wanted to move out of here. And so I was putting money away. Every time I got money, I was putting it away. . . . It just seems like everything goes great until something goes wrong.

One afternoon in March 2011, we talked about her housing options. I asked her about subsidized housing, and she shook her head:

Their waiting lists are so long. And with subsidy, they watch you so bad. . . . I applied for a place in Bradford [Vermont] and one in Randolph [Vermont]. Each one, you have to wait. They are so long, the waiting lists. I saw one in Hartford [Vermont], but it was eight years to get in there! It is so stupid. I don't know. I heard that it is kind of like you always have someone watching you and telling you what to do. They are nice apartments, but I just don't want anyone in my business all of the time, you know?

She was reluctantly considering moving back in with her best friend's family: "I don't really want to move out [there]. I will have like no life out there." She continued about other possibilities: "My mom wants me to move to Maine. But I really can't move to Maine. I don't know where I can go."

Over the next two months, Abigail moved multiple times, "couch surfing" with friends and acquaintances for a few days or weeks at a time. When we saw each other next, we met at a Dunkin' Donuts. Abigail picked at her glazed donut, her eyes downcast as she said, "I had a bad couple of weeks." She had shared an apartment with a friend, and then they moved in with some men for a few weeks where they were "partying all the time." Her children had stayed with family friends during this time. Now, Abigail was staying with her sister; Mary was with her father and Adam was with a family friend. Reflecting on her "bad couple of weeks," Abigail said she realized, "I just wasn't myself. I can't do this." Having experienced what she described as a "wake up call," Abigail was thinking about completing her GED and was considering joining Job Corps:

I'm doing this for my family. . . . I just look forward to the day when I can get a job. And welfare says that once I have a job, they will pay for daycare. If I could get a job for $10.50 an hour, I could live off that a lot better than I could live off welfare. I will figure something out. I usually do. I should work at McDonald's or something. I am so sick of welfare. I could just get a job. I want to work especially because my kids, they need daycare. . . . It would be nice. It would be really great.

But a few months later, things remained much the same, and Abigail and the kids had moved again, this time into an apartment with another family in the study: Nancy and her husband, Carl, and their two children. Like most doubling-up situations, the arrangement worked well for a while. The shared household allowed the adults to pool their resources and share responsibilities for childcare and housework.

But over time, relationships were strained, and, in this case, alliances shifted when Nancy's husband, Carl, had an affair with Abigail. Abigail had also recently learned that she was pregnant with her third child. She was unsure of who the father was, having had a series of brief sexual relationships with different men. Abigail and Carl moved out in the summer of 2011, and when I saw them next, they were staying with another friend. During this time, Abigail's children moved between staying with their fathers, family friends, and being with Abigail and Carl. When we met for lunch at a pizzeria, Carl was pale and wearing an ill-fitting t-shirt and torn jeans as he slid his rail-thin body across the booth. I asked how they were doing and Abigail responded immediately: "Tired." Carl added, "I really wanna get a place of our own. I'm sick of sleepin' on the couch." He looked at Abigail, "And I'm pretty sure you're sick of it, too. I wish we could find a two-bedroom house. I'm sick of livin' with other people." As we waited for our pizza, Carl counted out the cash in his pocket: $88. "We're basically broke," he said. He was recently fired from his job at a drycleaner and was hoping to land a job as a dishwasher.

In the fall of 2011, Abigail, Carl, and the children moved into Safe Harbor. This was Abigail's second stay at the shelter in a period of two years. During this time, she signed up for GED classes, and Carl was working long shifts as a hotel housekeeper. Staying at the shelter was helping them to save money: "All we are working on now is being able to find a place. We are saving up money to find a place and get out of here—once we get caught up on everything that we need to pay for. We're just a little bit behind from when I didn't have a job."

But this fragile stability was again shaken when they were asked to leave the shelter following an argument with another family. The shelter staff gave them a day to pack their belongings and agreed to pay for two nights at a nearby motel. Abigail was left with little more than a faint hope that she might get a break from a local nonprofit to help put a deposit on an apartment.

Not surprisingly, with their housing options dwindling in the Upper Valley, the couple made a decision to uproot the family and move out of state. This was a common narrative among other families I met. Southern states beckoned with the promise of cheaper housing and an escape from the harsh New England winter.

During their time in Georgia, Abigail fell out of touch with me, so I was surprised to hear about a year later in 2013 that she had returned to Vermont. She had broken up with Carl and wanted to be closer to her own family. She and the children were again living with her best friend's family but they spent much of their time with Nancy. The women had reconciled by this time, seemingly having bonded through a mutual dislike of Carl.

In early 2014, mirroring the gradual awakening of spring in New England—seen in melting snow banks and lengthening days—Abigail seemed poised for change. She had decided to take her mother's advice and move with her children to live with her parents in Maine. This move promised a way to escape the precarious cycles of mobility that had marked Abigail's experience for over four years: "I have realized I'm only good for these people for my rent and cleaning their house. I just can't wait to move to Maine." The anticipation of the move appeared to catalyze something bigger within Abigail. She articulated an active striving toward greater well-being in a post she shared with me: "Making new changes to my life, hopefully for the good. For my health, I want to start eating healthier and try and quit smoking. For my mental health, I have started cutting out the bad people in my life that have seemed to bring me down. Looking forward to a better, healthier life."

My last visit with Abigail was as she packed up boxes, preparing for the move. She had recently reunited with her youngest son, who had been living with her parents in Maine. Her mood turned reflective:

> I would say the biggest thing that means the most to me is my family and my kids. They are always the ones by my side through thick and thin. They will be there with open arms, no matter how bad I mess up. . . . When my parents got here with [my youngest son], he was just getting out of the car and couldn't see me. But when he did, he started crying, ran over, and said, "My mama, my mama," and he gave me a big hug. It's the little things in life that mean the most to me.

Nancy

In the spring of 2010, with her prospects of landing subsidized housing remote, Nancy and her toddler-age daughter, Emily, moved from Safe Harbor into a two-bedroom townhouse where they doubled up with a couple who were friends of Nancy's. Nancy was in her mid-20s at this time, White, and pregnant with her second child. Soon after moving, her son, David, was born, and Nancy reunited with David's father, Carl. They were married that summer in a small backyard ceremony. The townhouse was bursting at the seams with four adults, a toddler, and a newborn under its roof. Nevertheless, Nancy was grateful to be out of the shelter, and, for a time, the shared household provided much needed support.

Yet as spring turned into summer, the convivial atmosphere turned tense, and the friendships began to fray. The townhouse, which had been a collective source of pride, became increasingly messy: food-encrusted dishes were stacked in the sink, garbage bags were left overflowing in the kitchen, empty soda cans and potato chip bags were scattered in the living room. Chores that had once been shared became the source of finger pointing ("It's *her turn* to do the dishes").

Then on August 30, 2010, I received the following text message: "We r being evicted and are going to a motel." Nancy's friends, who held the lease, had neglected to pay the rent for several months. Nancy, Carl, Emily, and David moved into a pay-by-the-week motel, where they stayed for four months.

Two weeks before Christmas 2010, the family moved again, this time into a two-bedroom apartment of their own. Beaming with pride, Nancy gave me a tour. For the first time in her life, Emily had her own room. A few months later, with money from their tax refund, the couple furnished the apartment with items from Walmart and Rent-a-Center. The balance of the refund went to advance rent payments. With relief resonating in her voice, Nancy said, "We're paid through April." With income from Carl's job at a drycleaner supplemented by SNAP benefits and occasional contributions from couch-surfing friends, the family's financial situation was tight, but they managed to make ends meet.

But this fragile stability was upended two weeks shy of their one-year anniversary when Carl declared he wanted a divorce in the midst of an affair with Abigail. With divorce imminent, Nancy navigated not only deep betrayal ("The girl who's supposed to be my best friend steals my husband") but also the loss of steady income from Carl's job and, consequently, her housing security: "I'll probably be homeless again." With financial help from her parents to continue paying the $800 monthly market-rate rent, Nancy and her children held onto the apartment for two years following her divorce.

Ultimately, Nancy's parents were unable to continue paying the rent indefinitely, and the young family again faced homelessness. Nancy and her children moved five times in the following year. After losing the apartment, they took refuge at a family shelter in a distant part of New Hampshire. From there, they moved into a pay-by-the-week motel, where they stayed for two months. Unlike "Heroin Hotel," where many families stayed at various points throughout the research, this establishment had a "nice" reputation. One sticky late spring day as we visited, Nancy propped open the room door to let in fresh air and sunshine. We sat on the two queen beds eating our lunch of McDonald's hamburgers and watched her two small children wielding their plastic Happy Meal treasures. My attention gradually shifted from the children's busyness inside the room to a growing awareness of feeling surveilled by the middle-aged male motel owner outside the room. Treading slowly like a cop on the beat, he repeatedly passed by the room's open door as he tried to discern the nature of our interaction.

After two months, the family was forced to move out of the motel in anticipation of the different clientele that would be brought by the local college's graduation and the summer tourism season. Nancy once again packed up their belongings and returned for her second stint at "Heroin Hotel." A few weeks later, she was informed that she would need to move out immediately because she had stayed for 28 days. She explained that after 28 days people qualified as "tenants" in Vermont. Thus, motel owners routinely required residents to move out for a few days to avoid the possibility of residents invoking tenants' rights. Looking around at the crates and garbage bags that held her family's possessions, Nancy heaved a deep sigh: "How the hell am I supposed to pack all this up by myself?"

From the motel, Nancy and the children doubled up with another family in a cramped apartment for two months before moving to an apartment of their own in a small Vermont town. They lived in this apartment for nine months spanning 2013 and 2014. Here, they once again settled into the routines of domestic life. Emily started kindergarten here. The small village school seemed to offer Emily a refuge from the challenges of her home life. As Nancy explained: "She doesn't like the weekends. She wants to go back to school." Nancy had enrolled in online classes—hoping one day to become a daycare provider. She voiced her awareness of the limits she faced with low-wage work: "I'll be 30 in November. That's also the reason I want to go back to school and everything. I'll turn 30, I have two kids, and I'm doing it all by myself. And it's, like, I can't get anything better than a crummy cashiering job or, you know, a fast-food job or anything that pays like crap."

Yet over time she found it increasingly difficult to balance her schoolwork and caregiving responsibilities. During this time, the family survived on cash benefits from Vermont, SNAP benefits, and the Special Supplemental Nutrition Program for Women, Infants, and Children (WIC). One afternoon after running errands at a Walmart 30 miles away, our conversation turned to money. Knowing that the bulk of her cash benefits went to paying for her market-rate apartment, I asked how much she had left over after paying rent: it was $84. Nancy relied on drips and drabs of financial support from her mother, who would step in to pay for diapers or for food when it inevitably ran low at the end of the month. Nancy reciprocated when she could with small gifts—an anniversary card, photographs of the children, drugstore trinkets announcing in curly scroll, "Family is forever."

With over 90% of her cash benefits going to rent, I was not surprised when an old acquaintance moved in. He contributed to the household by buying cigarettes for Nancy and giving her access to a car—a lifeline in a rural town with no public transportation. Nancy was grateful for the transportation and for the comfort of having someone around. For several months, this arrangement provided a sense of stability and security for Nancy and her children. Yet the fragility of this arrangement was apparent when Nancy later clarified the nature of their relationship: "He's not my boyfriend, but we're sleeping together."

Six months after he moved out, Nancy was again facing eviction after falling behind on rent. With no prospects for a place she could afford in Vermont at the time, Nancy took an impromptu offer from the mother of a childhood friend to move south. Remarkably, after learning of Nancy's plight on Facebook, the woman drove through the night to pick up Nancy and the children, loaded what they could fit into her truck, and drove back to Georgia: "Mama wasn't going to let those babies be on the street."

A year later, in the summer of 2015, Nancy and the children moved back to Vermont. They had become homeless again in Georgia. Upon returning to Vermont, Nancy reconnected with her case manager, Jamie, from Safe Harbor. As is detailed in chapter 6, this marked a moment that would change this family's trajectory through access to subsidized housing.

Episodic Homelessness, Chronic Housing Insecurity

Taking a long view of families' trajectories provides insight into what happens to families in the community following a period of homelessness. Over time, families experienced periods of both relative security and urgency with their housing situations. Abigail moved 14 times between March 2010, when she was a guest at Safe Harbor, and June 2014, when she moved out of state to live with her parents. Her decision to leave the subsidized apartment following her stay at Safe Harbor was momentous: she lost her housing subsidy. This sparked a cycle of continued mobility for Abigail and her children as she sought access to affordable housing in a rural setting marked by shortages of housing stock. This mirrors Nancy's experience of moving 11 times between leaving Safe Harbor in March 2010 and moving into her first subsidized apartment in August 2015. Both of these young women spent years moving between tenuous arrangements of doubling up, long stretches in shabby motels, brief returns to homeless shelters, as well as periods of fragile security.

Whereas homelessness is episodic, all but one family in the study endured chronic housing insecurity in the years following their initial stay at Safe Harbor (see the appendix for family housing trajectories). Families continued to live "on the edge" of losing housing, and the specter of homelessness loomed large in their lived experiences. In rural New England, families' survival was often predicated on finding what leaders at Safe Harbor described as "shelter but not housing," with frequent moves among sympathetic or exploitive associates of closer or more tangential relationships. These families existed "on the edge" of homelessness, with mobility becoming a paradoxical constant in their lives. Throughout the study, families lost housing for a range of reasons, including disputes with landlords, child custody issues, divorce, and an inability to afford rent. With few options available for affordable housing, when families experienced a housing crisis, they commonly turned to friends or family for temporary shelter. Taking in roommates and "crashing" with others was common practice, especially among young parents. This reflected a collective reciprocity whereby, during times of greater stability, families would frequently host others on their couches or floors. When I visited with families, I would routinely meet new people who were staying for a few days in exchange for a small contribution to rent, groceries, babysitting, or cigarettes. Then, in their own times of need, some families would reach out to those in their networks to find a place to stay. "Doubling up" was understood as a temporary strategy, and these informal living arrangements were precarious as the stresses of overcrowding, divergent parenting styles, and different housekeeping standards took their toll.

Motels often served as stop-gap housing when families had exhausted their "couch surfing" privileges. Four of the five families lived for long stretches, typically months at a time, in motels over the course of the research. Motels were viewed as an unpleasant option, and participants expressed concerns about their families' health and safety in these settings where they were at the mercy of the rules (and whims) of motel owners. Although frequently in disrepair, motels were a costly option. In some cases, families met the rigid eligibility criteria for access to motel vouchers from the state of Vermont. But more frequently, families drew on cash benefits or wages to pay for rooms that cost over $1,000 per month. Families were keenly aware of the cruel reality of paying roughly the equivalent of a market-rate apartment for a worn-out room with a microwave and mini-fridge and a backdrop of daily worry over drug activity and violence. Yet they remained caught in a cycle of overpaying by the week because of the impossibility of saving enough on service-sector wages for a security deposit plus first and last months' rent.

Despite their serious drawbacks, motels nevertheless served a critical role in the housing landscape in rural New England as a low-barrier way to access shelter during a time of crisis because individuals needed only to come up with the cash for a night or a week. In a setting marked by serious housing shortages and few congregate family shelters, motels became a lifeline for families that had run out of options for a roof and a bed. In the absence of motels, families in the study would have contended with the harsher realities of procuring shelter through more distant people in their social networks or faced literal homelessness and the prospect of "camping" outdoors or sleeping in cars.

Once housed, out-of-pocket housing expenses dominated families' budgets for those without access to subsidies. In this northern climate, families also faced the high cost of heating homes during the long winter, a situation commonly exacerbated by old, energy-inefficient housing. Families cobbled together resources from wage work and benefits, the generosity of family members, or contributions from friends who doubled up with them. For periods of time, these arrangements allowed some families to gain access to market-rate housing. But an eventual disruption loomed on every family's horizon that revealed the fragility of their hard-won and creative braiding of resources. These disruptions took different forms—an unexpected car repair, an illness leading to a lost job, a strained marriage reaching its breaking point, the accretion of the daily expenses of raising a family. None of the families in the study were able to sustain paying market-rate rents on their own, and they found themselves packing up belongings again and again for yet another move.

"We're Not 'Making It,' but We're Trying": Money and Work in Rural New England

Consistent with evidence demonstrating that the majority of participants in public support programs such as Temporary Aid to Needy Families (TANF) and the Supplemental Nutrition Assistance Program (SNAP) are members of working families (Allegretto et al., 2013), all households in the study had adults employed at various points over the course of the research. Mothers with infants and toddlers typically took time away from the workforce during their children's early years and relied on cash benefit support from TANF as well as food assistance through SNAP and the Special Supplemental Nutrition Program for Women, Infants, and Children (WIC) program. In some cases, mothers worked informally babysitting for others or cleaning houses for cash, but opportunities for informal work were limited by a lack of childcare and lack of transportation. Once children were regularly attending school, parents reentered the workforce, most often in low-wage service-sector jobs. Yet gaps in work histories posed challenges for finding jobs among some parents when they were ready to transition from full-time caregiving to paid work, as Nancy explained when her youngest was beginning preschool: "I haven't worked in four years. So that's another thing being held against me."

Parents held jobs in a variety of service and retail settings—grocery stores, pharmacies, dollar stores, gas stations, and big box stores. These positions were part-time, had no health insurance or other benefits, and had unpredictable work schedules. Parents were at the mercy of managers and the whims of robo-scheduling. Working parents rarely knew their schedules more than a week in advance. For single mothers, such uncertainty posed an ongoing tension with the demands of caregiving for their young children. Some parents, like Nancy, leveraged networks of friends and neighbors that enabled access to just-in-time childcare on evenings or weekends. But such arrangements would eventually—seemingly inevitably—fray, leading parents to leave one job in search of another one with the promise of more favorable hours.

Others cycled through jobs for different reasons. Nancy's husband, Carl, was fired from his job at a drycleaner when he did not show up for work after contracting the flu. His boss refused to grant him sick days. Some quit jobs after feeling "disrespected" by supervisors or growing frustrated with "slacking" coworkers, as was the case with Barbara, who left numerous jobs over the course of the study.

Job prospects were limited for those without access to a vehicle or who lived far from a bus line. Barbara and her long-term partner shared one vehicle, and she explained how limited transportation and long travel distances impacted her ability to work. After they moved into an apartment in a small town in New Hampshire, she stated:

> I am hoping that this summer, I am going to check this little town out. I want to just get a little job there. I don't want something that I am going to have to travel to. You know. We only have one car. And that is kind of what stops me from working. It is because, you know [pause]. It is not that I don't want to work because I do. If I could find something I could walk to—or I could take the bike. Because the job I am thinking of, you are not going to make a million dollars, anyway, okay? And, you know, to put everything out for gas is ridiculous.

Some towns in the Upper Valley are served by a free bus service, but this public transportation is geographically limited to the population centers of the region and runs only during daytime hours on weekdays, limiting its usefulness for those working shifts in the evening or on weekends. Among families with cars, their vehicles were old and unreliable. When Tara's truck broke down and needed costly repairs that she could not afford, she was unable to continue her job as a supermarket cashier. Similarly, Carl quit another job when his van "blew up." He described calling "everyone I know who lives even remotely close to us" to get a ride to work. But "They told me that by the time I paid gas money, I wouldn't have nothin' left in my check. It's not worth it, they told me." Cycling through jobs in this fashion meant that working parents were not positioned to experience benefits that may come with greater job seniority, and they were often unable to draw on previous employers for positive references.

Despite these challenges and the often difficult nature of low-wage service jobs, parents valued work. One summer afternoon, Abigail and I were catching up over iced coffee at Dunkin' Donuts. As tiny rivers of condensation made their way down our plastic cups, she told me that she had been working with vocational rehabilitation services to make a plan to complete the final two credits needed for her high school degree. She hoped that her job prospects would improve once she had her degree in hand.

For Abigail and others, getting a job was about much more than simply a paycheck. Imagining her life with a job, it became clear that work was a powerful symbol of capability and self-sufficiency to Abigail as a young mother: "I wanna prove to her [a family friend] that I *can* support two kids. All I gotta do is get a job. I *really* need to get a job." Likewise, during a period of unemployment, Nancy longed for the structure and sense of purpose her previous job at the dollar store had provided. Barbara expressed a similar sentiment when she said, "You always feel better when you're working and doing something productive." After cycling through jobs as a hotel housekeeper, a cashier at a bus station convenience store, and a clerk at a drycleaner, Barbara was thrilled when she was finally able to apply her training as a medical assistant when she found a job as a nursing aide at an assisted living facility. In her previous positions, she had longed for a job "where there is some kind of reward other than a few pennies in my pocket." Despite the difficult work of intimate care for elders—bathing, feeding, changing diapers—Barbara found value and meaning in this work: "I really feel like I'm doing God's work. I just look at it as caring for someone's loved one." These experiences illuminate that in the context of the deep stigma associated with poverty, work was both an opportunity for repairing the failures of homelessness and for expressing one's worthiness (cf. Snell-Rood & Carpenter-Song, 2018) and alignment with the New England bootstrap mentality.

Money, like jobs, tended to come and go among the families in the study. At one point, Barbara confided that she had always struggled with managing money: "As soon as I have it, it's gone." For some families, infusions of cash—from paychecks, tax refunds, or birthday and Christmas gifts—were met with a spirit of celebration and enabled them to make advance payments on rent or to purchase a used car. Among others, such cash infusions would be quickly spent on self-described splurges ranging from modest purchases such as toys or a new blanket from Walmart to larger purchases of televisions, computers, or furniture from Rent-a-Center.

Although conservative discourse often maligns such patterns of spending as irresponsible, a view grounded in the lived experiences of families surviving in poverty and attuned to broader cultural patterns offers fundamentally different interpretations. First, parents were deeply aware of the paradox of low-wage work. As Nancy stated wryly: "We're not 'making it,' but we're trying. You can work 40 hours a week and still not 'make it' these days. It's crazy." Through this lens, infusions of cash resources offered families rare opportunities to experience the psychological and social benefits of having a financial cushion—experiences that were typically out of reach despite their hard work.

Second, families were also aware of limits on their accrual of resources in the context of government benefits. For example, a family of three receiving Financial Assistance to Needy Families (FANF) in New Hampshire could have a maximum monthly income of $1,098 and no more than $2,000 in assets (New Hampshire Bureau of Family Assistance, 2021). Working parents would typically decline opportunities for promotions or more hours due to the risk that greater resources would jeopardize their access to Medicaid and other benefits. Over the course of the study, many who had "worked too much" experienced having their SNAP benefits substantially reduced or cut off for periods of time. Rigid benefit eligibility rules were a serious disincentive to saving additional resources.

In addition, spending—rather than saving—is culturally normative behavior in the United States. As such, spending down resources demonstrates that despite living "on the edge," parents nonetheless ascribed to and participated in mainstream values and practices in the U.S. Yet this has serious consequences for the ability to weather financial stresses, as a 2019 Federal Reserve report found that approximately 40% of U.S. adults would have difficulty covering an unexpected expense of $400 (Federal Reserve, 2019).

Finally, living in poverty often meant that families overpaid for basic necessities—transportation, access to a motel room, higher-priced food at a convenience store within walking distance. Underscoring this reality, Jim described an exchange he had with a child welfare worker:

> Do you know how much it costs for a cab? We have to pay for a cab if we wanna go to the store. Cabs and, before we got into this house, hotel rooms. I just said [to the case worker], "You're not looking at this realistically. None of you people have been in our position. You don't know what it *costs* to be homeless. Unless we wanna sleep on the street!"

In the context of trying but not making it, families endured conditions of extreme scarcity on a regular basis. Parents in the study often preferred to schedule our ethnographic visits toward the end of the month so the modest research stipend could help bridge expenses before paychecks or the next month's benefits became available. During one visit, Nancy stated, "I hate the end of the month," and invited me to look through her kitchen cabinets, which were sparsely stocked with a few canned goods and packages of noodles. I opened her refrigerator and found only a pound of ground beef, a loaf of bread, and a gallon of milk. Most months, Nancy would appeal to her mother to buy household basics and personal care items (such as toilet paper, soap, and sanitary pads) that were not eligible expenses under SNAP rules.

With the help of case managers and the advice of friends, families grew knowledgeable about how to procure a range of material resources. Families benefitted from the robust nonprofit sector in the region to gain access to food, clothing, and used furniture as well as access to subsidies such as heating assistance. In addition, informal networks of exchange were also common. As I describe above in relation to doubling up, such networks could facilitate access to immediate needs—a ride, a few cigarettes, toilet paper. Nancy cultivated a broad group of friends and associates and invested in these relationships by providing others with a couch to sleep on, childcare, or small gifts when she could. Yet such networks were also often fragile and unpredictable. As detailed in their family portraits, both Nancy and Abigail experienced deeply uneven exchanges over the years that ultimately resulted in another housing crisis for both of their families.

Isolation in Rural New England

Long travel distances and limited means of public transportation in rural New England communities made it challenging to access resources and accomplish basic household tasks such as shopping for groceries or doing laundry. One summer afternoon, surrounded by boxes of fresh produce and bags of groceries, Jim recounted his 80-mile route to food pantries in several small towns in the Upper Valley. He estimated the trip took him three hours: "It takes a lot of time—takes a lot of gas." For Jim, the time, effort, and money he spent on the trip were worth it to gain access to a wider variety of foods than the shelf-stable and processed fare more readily available. Some families that did not own a car found themselves walking long distances along rural roads with narrow shoulders and no sidewalks. Barbara remembered her experiences as a young mother walking to the grocery store:

> I remember not having a car and trying to get to the grocery store, and it was winter. And—oh, my god—and by the time I got—we had a backpack this big [gestures wide with her hands]. And my son I was carrying on one side, and I was carrying the groceries on the other. Oh, my god. But, you know, you got to do what you got to do. Either that or we weren't going to eat.

Others relied on rides from friends or family members, which required careful coordination and planning ahead for scheduled school or doctor's appointments. For many families, grocery shopping involved a daylong outing to stock up on essentials at grocery stores, Walmart, and discount warehouse stores. Accompanying Nancy on some of these trips, I noticed her preferences for canned and prepackaged goods that were shelf-stable as she loaded the two carts that were filled by the end of her shopping. This was a common strategy as parents sought to collect several weeks' worth of food and supplies at once in the absence of access to regular transportation. Standing in the checkout line with Nancy, I was keenly aware of the judgmental gaze of fellow shoppers as their eyes scanned the heaping contents of her carts.

Living at a distance from town centers, with limited or no means of transportation, many in the study contended with isolation in this rural context. As families sought access to more affordable housing options, many moved to geographically remote towns in the region. Their initial elation at finding housing was often quickly tempered by the reality of finding themselves alone and tending to young children far from family and friends. Over the years, I observed how geographic and social isolation intertwined to render families vulnerable to unhealthy relationships, self-defeating decisions, and mental health and substance use challenges. As detailed in her family portrait, Abigail sacrificed the security of a subsidized apartment for the promise of relief from loneliness. In Nancy's experience, taking in an old acquaintance gave her access to a car that broke the grinding isolation and inconveniences of life without transportation in a small, rural town. Yet Nancy's desire for companionship and need for transportation (she had neither a driver's license nor a car) led her to accept highly unequal terms of doubling up in exchange for rides and cigarettes. She attributed her ongoing struggles with anxiety with "being by myself with the kids for so long" in this remote town.

For Tara, another young mother in the study, her fragile sobriety was continually tested by the loneliness and boredom she felt in her rural apartment: "There's nothing to do here. . . . I don't have any friends. The only people I talk to are from the state." Despite her desire to distance herself from the "losers" in her life, Tara was ultimately drawn back into the network of drug users in her small town. Hannah also commonly stated that she "has no one else to talk to" and "no one to ask" for small favors like a ride to the grocery store or to a doctor's appointment. In fact, when I offered to give her a ride one evening to pick up supplies in anticipation of a snowstorm, it seemed that Hannah had given up on the possibility of such small acts of kindness. Hannah's response to my offer was poignant: "Nobody's ever asked that. I don't know what to say."

Precarity of Relationships

The sense of isolation felt by many in the study also reflected the precarity of relationships. Over time, I observed a rhythm of social ties being created, tested, and often broken. Steady friendships were rare. As discussed in chapter 2, relationships with extended family were fraught for many in the study. When Tara moved out of Safe Harbor and back to her hometown in Vermont, she was disappointed by the lack of support from her parents:

> I really thought I was gonna have my family's support living here. I really did. Me and my dad used to be really close. . . . He never came anywhere. Never came to [the shelter]. You know what I mean? I've been in [hometown] almost two—how long have I been here? Two months? Going on two months? Never came.

For the young women in the study—Abigail, Nancy, and Tara—their relationships with romantic partners seemed especially fragile. Abigail had children with three different men. She shared custody of her daughter, Mary, which brought complications in terms of different parenting styles and expectations for care. At one point, Mary had an ongoing problem with head lice, which her father had neglected to treat. Despite sharing custody, Abigail appeared to expect very little from her former boyfriend: "I thought that people changed when they had kids. I guess girls change, but guys don't." Abigail explained to me that she found it easier with her middle child, Adam, because she had sole custody: "It's easy because he is *my* kid. It is like his father doesn't want to have anything to do with him." The father of her youngest child was in jail and was uninvolved in parenting. While, in some cases, single parenting may have reduced conflict, women were nonetheless left to shoulder both the responsibility and expense of raising of a family. Many of the women in the study were owed substantial amounts from former partners for child support.

Tara was married but had an on-again-off-again relationship with her husband, Chris. Similar to the limited parenting involvement of Abigail's former boyfriend, one afternoon Tara and I returned from running errands together. Chris had been watching their toddler son while we were out. Shoes and toys were scattered across the floor of the living room. Scooping up her son, Tara said with exasperation, "You had fun, didn't you?" Then her attention turned to the child's sagging diaper. "When was the last time that you changed him?" she asked Chris, shaking her head. "God, Chris, how many hours has it been?" She whisked her son upstairs to change him, and I overheard her say in a singsong voice crisp with resentment, "Daddy doesn't like to change your diapers." Later, after Chris had left, Tara told me that this was the first time that Chris had watched their son for longer than an hour. A few months later, when Tara was pregnant with their second child, Chris's unreliability had sharpened into seeming indifference:

> He knows that I am pregnant. And he knows everything that is going on, but he doesn't want anything to do with me. And it is really upsetting me. And I am, like, you need to come to the doctor with me or something. I got the [ultrasound] pictures back. He didn't even care. You know what I mean?

With arguments escalating between them, Tara applied for and received a restraining order:

> [Chris] was just being a jerk, and he would pop by whenever, and [pause] I don't know. He tried kicking the door in one day. He was—breaking in and stealing my key. Stupid shit. So I had to get a, I had to get a res—I had to get a "no-trespassing allowed." There's so many ups and downs with us, you know what I mean? I want our home to feel safe to [my son]. Not a battleground, you know what I mean?

Tara eventually filed for divorce.

Among other families, spouses and long-term partnerships were a substantial source of support in the midst of the daily onslaught of insecurity. Yet even steady relationships were made fragile by the struggles of everyday life. Following the removal of their children by the Vermont Department of Children and Families, Jim and Hannah struggled to secure stable housing, a condition for being reunited with their children. When their landlord refused to make home repairs that were required to meet Section 8 standards, the couple found themselves homeless again. During this time, after two months of living in a tent, with the New England late summer nights growing steadily cooler, the strain of homelessness took a toll on this long-married couple. They separated for several weeks when Hannah hitched a ride to a town three hours north with the prospect of a place to stay with an acquaintance. Jim "crashed" during this time with a young woman. Jim and Hannah eventually reconciled and reunited, but other couples were not as fortunate. I remember being shocked by the suddenness of Carl's announcement that he wanted to divorce Nancy just two weeks shy of their one-year wedding anniversary. Only a few weeks before, Nancy had been imagining a future vacation after Carl had worked long enough to earn paid time off.

Enduring at the Margins: Striving for Ordinary

In this chapter, I have focused on the myriad threats to stability faced by families in the study—chronic housing insecurity, challenging low-wage work, extreme financial scarcity, profound isolation in rural communities, and precarious relationships. These experiences form a backdrop of *fundamental insecurity* in the lives of families that lays bare the fragility of life on the edge. The constellation of social and structural vulnerabilities constrains opportunities to make it in this setting and creates pressures within interpersonal relationships that further limit stability. Yet even as these profound social and economic forces shape and constrain families' opportunities, close attention to lived experience reveals the specific strategies and actions that enable families to endure. How do these families endure at the margins, living with profound scarcity of material resources in a context of abundance, bearing intense loneliness wrought by rejection and isolation within small-town communities? How does family life endure in the midst of shame and feelings of failure as a mother or father?

Despite being profoundly marginalized, all families in the study longed for and made efforts toward living "ordinary" lives. The ordinary evokes everyday life as unremarkable, the stuff of commonplace routines, the quotidian and mundane. As anthropological scholars have observed, however, this sense of the ordinary brings with it a deeply ethical bearing reflective of normative values and cultural orientations (Lambek, 2010; Mattingly, 2018). In the context of Northern New England, ordinary family life is marked by the presence of material, personal, and social resources—having a home of one's own, enough money for necessities and some niceties, and time and resources to participate in family and community activities. For families surviving in poverty in this setting, these signifiers of the good life are largely out of reach (Mattingly, 2014). Yet as I observed over time, families *strive* for the ordinary amid lives marked by fundamental insecurity.

For some, this was brought forth in the imaginal space of memory and desire. One late winter afternoon, Nancy and I sat together in the living room of her apartment. Reaching over to a small table beside the couch, she lifted a stack of photo albums. "Did I ever show you these?" she asked. "These are my scrapbooks." As she opened the first album, I scooted closer to her on the couch for a better look. For nearly an hour, she slowly guided me through the pages, beginning with her baby pictures and ending in her high school years. The fading photographs were surrounded by colorful construction paper borders with handwritten captions in her bubbly print. I found myself painfully aware of the disjunction between the smiling faces, the eyes shining with pride and hope, and my knowledge of Nancy's frayed relationships with her family. As she showed me a photograph of her modest childhood home, I wondered if she was thinking of when she had been "kicked out" as a teenager or, more recently, when she felt that she and her infant daughter would place too many demands for space and resources to be taken in when they lost their housing.

Yet as she reverently turned the pages of the albums in the blue glow of her television, I realized that these photographs pointed to family life as Nancy wished to remember it. In much the same way, prior to her divorce Nancy proudly declared herself "married with two kids" whenever she ran into old friends and acquaintances. Her words conjured a 1950s domestic tableau that belied the harsh reality of life in a cramped, dark apartment smelling forever of cigarette smoke, dirty diapers, and a cat box; a place where the cupboards became scarce at the end of every month and the walls contained the raised voices and slammed doors of the arguments between Nancy and her husband.

Striving for ordinary was manifest in small actions and subtle ways. When living in motels, parents always personalized these spaces with small signifiers of home by displaying photographs or using their own bed linens. After losing her apartment, Tara seemed to find momentary solace in buying herself nail polish at the drugstore. As I watched her trace her fingers slowly across the small glass bottles, the globes of glittery color appeared to transport her, however briefly, away from the harsh reality of homelessness and loss. Parents shielded their children from the knowledge of their precarious finances with celebrations of birthdays and holidays. Nancy created holiday traditions; every Christmas, the children received a new ornament. Each year when Nancy put up their Christmas tree, she would call my attention to this family archive, and we would marvel together at the passing of time as she pointed out the shiny ornaments decorated with Disney princesses and superheroes. Even when Tara had no money with which to buy birthday presents for her four-year-old son, she baked a cake, decorated the apartment with colorful balloons, and made a large "Happy Birthday!" banner. Others concealed (or denied) the gravity of their economic situations by engaging in celebratory spending of infusions of cash.

Families also expressed their desires for an ordinary life in the aftermath of homelessness through the mundane activities of keeping house. After a period of homelessness, having an apartment or a house of one's own appeared to take on heightened significance, and, for some, domestic tasks became a way of rooting oneself to a new place. Jim took great pride in cultivating a vast organic vegetable garden. During the summer months, he and Hannah would send me off with fresh greens and zucchini after our visits. Barbara enjoyed keeping a "spotless" house. When we ran errands together, she would often stock up on purple jugs of sweetly fragranced cleaning fluid. Nancy honed her cooking skills and developed a repertoire of dishes for her family. She was known for her pork tenderloin and crock-pot chicken and noodles; these were frequent requests among friends visiting or "crashing" for the night.

Even in the face of seemingly insurmountable challenges, families continued to hope for and make efforts toward a better future. For some, this manifested in concerted efforts to find a job or return to school. The frequent changing of jobs observed over time reflects parents' efforts to improve their working conditions in the context of the difficult and often unforgiving nature of service-sector work. Parents were deeply aware of the limits they faced with low-wage work and hoped their children would find other opportunities. Barbara advised her teenage children: "I tell them the doors will fly open if they get an education. Otherwise, they're going to have meager wages for the rest of their lives." Some found solace and hope for the future in religion. Barbara read the bible and listened to Christian ministers on the radio every morning, holding fast to her conviction that God has a plan for her family and that her children will learn from her own mistakes. For others, connections to family and caring for children served as moorings amid uncertainty.

Families endure, at least in part, through their participation in small, restorative rituals that bind them to the rhythms of a more secure domestic life. Writing about recovery in the aftermath of collective trauma, Veena Das and Arthur Kleinman (2001) note that "in relation to lives severely disrupted, to be able to secure the everyday life by individuals and communities is indeed an achievement" (p. 1). What appears prosaic takes on deep significance in the aftermath of the loss of home and social ties and assaults on identity. Encapsulated in the minutiae of daily life—keeping house, making dinner, looking at family photos—are families' intense desires for and efforts toward ordinary lives unmarked by the stigma of homelessness and the grind of life on the edge. Writing about the "terrifying nightmares" of serious illness or tragedy, Cheryl Mattingly (2010) notes that families engage in "work to make them habitable, to find within their terrifying terrain quieter moments, even small lush pleasures" (p. 4).

Families resist the demoralization of not being able to make it in a context in which self-sufficiency is prized by striving to adhere to local community norms, including self-sufficiency and rugged individualism (Fitchen, 1991; Lawrence, 1995; Sherman, 2006; Wagner et al., 1995). On the one hand, these efforts may be a balm for the wounds of social defeat (Marrow & Luhrmann, 2012). On the other hand, families are also reinforcing the New England bootstrap mentality in ways that may be self-defeating. Withdrawing from social contact to protect against gossip and humiliation may worsen families' isolation and loneliness. Engaging in heavy consumer spending may allow one to save face but also renders families in precarious financial circumstances even more economically vulnerable. Young women may be especially vulnerable to being taken advantage of as they struggle to meet their families' basic needs.

Amid the conditions of fundamental insecurity, families engaged in daily struggle (Jenkins, 2015b; Jenkins & Csordas, 2020), creatively and imperfectly improvising strategies enabling their survival. The efforts of families as they strive for ordinary offer a powerful counternarrative to prevailing cultural discourses of deficit and stigma. Close attention to the lives of families creates opportunities to recognize the profound precarity they experience while also illuminating the strengths and resourcefulness of families marginalized by poverty and housing insecurity.

4 Paradoxes of Care

In the crisis and aftermath of homelessness, the lives of the families in this study were subsumed by *fundamental insecurity*. As detailed in the previous chapter, a housing crisis is an acute experience—being evicted by landlords, getting kicked out by friends, not knowing where your family will spend the night. But the crisis that eventuates in homelessness for families is part of a longer horizon of experience marked by instability, impermanence, and mobility (cf. Vissing, 1996). Against this backdrop, the families in the study interacted regularly with organizations and institutions as part of their daily efforts to meet basic needs. Unlike many rural communities, the Upper Valley is a resource-rich environment: the region is home to an academic medical center as well as a vast collection of healthcare organizations and nonprofit social service providers. In this landscape, families were entangled in a kaleidoscope of professional services—housing and social services, mental health and substance use treatment, legal services, and the child welfare system. And yet the presence and availability of systems and institutions often did not translate into robust and sustained supports for families. Despite struggling with chronic physical health, mental health, and substance use challenges in the context of living in poverty, over time it became clear that most families remained quite tenuously and haphazardly engaged with professional services.

This chapter focuses on these *paradoxes of care* to explore the troubled interface between marginalized rural families, care providers, and the systems of care intended to support families. Although many of my interlocuters often sharply critiqued institutions of care, their views of services were dynamic and open to change. While past negative experiences could make people reluctant to seek care and could shape expectations of poor treatment by providers, trusted relationships did exist and were cultivated under some conditions. Health and social service providers that value and incorporate knowledge of the conditions of fundamental insecurity can create opportunities for shifts in how families engage in care, a theme that is elaborated in chapter 6. In this chapter, I focus on patterns of engagement that reflect missed opportunities within institutions of care to more fully support those on the margins.

In documenting how families navigate through the complex landscape of care in rural New England, I situate this endeavor within decades of research in anthropology and cultural psychiatry examining tensions between clinical and community orientations to suffering. This body of scholarship illuminates the diverse ways in which problems are identified, conceptualized, and explained. The personal and cultural meanings of suffering influence decisions by individuals and families about whether to seek help and what forms of help are considered appropriate. Biomedical and "psy-" renderings of forms of suffering are but one lens of understanding. Problems that may be diagnosable as mental illnesses can be understood as arising from chemical imbalances, stress and trauma, interpersonal conflict, personal moral failure, or supernatural causes (Carpenter-Song et al., 2010; Jenkins, 1988; Jenkins & Barrett, 2004). Moreover, anthropologists have provided insight into questions of why individuals with mental illness may still opt out of participating in mental health and social services. In her ethnographic research among women experiencing psychosis and homelessness in Chicago, Tanya Luhrmann (2008) found that women's refusal of housing services was an assertion of "competence and strength in a social setting in which those attributes are highly valued" (p. 19). This interpretation aligns with Kim Hopper's (2006) argument that refusal of services by marginalized people "may well be one of the last exercises of self-respect available to the conventionally powerless" (p. 219).

The misalignment between biomedical and individual, familial, and community perspectives may account, in part, for why the majority of people with mental health problems in the United States do not seek professional treatment (Wang et al., 2005). Within the context of mental health and substance use, the paradoxes that I have observed among families in the study reflect broader epidemiological patterns that consistently demonstrate that the majority of those with mental health and substance use challenges in the U.S. do not receive treatment (Ali et al., 2015; Wang et al., 2005). This treatment gap is an enduring conundrum for mental health services researchers, policy makers, and healthcare providers. The gap appears to be worse in rural areas of the U.S. Despite higher rates of depression (Hauenstein & Peddada, 2007) and suicide (Hirsch & Cukrowicz, 2014) and substance use rates equal to urban areas (Dew et al., 2007), rural populations are less likely to receive treatment compared to their urban counterparts (Wang et al., 2005).

Beyond considerations of diverse orientations to suffering, paradoxes of care also necessitate engagement with the culture of biomedicine and psychiatry. Scholarship in medical anthropology and social medicine has long critiqued biomedicine's reductive potential and emphasis on efficiency (Engel, 1977; B. Good, 1994; Kleinman, 1995; Mishler, 1981) that create conditions for eliding suffering through inattention to complex social problems. The consequences of the systemic sidelining of suffering are manifest in the persistent health inequities borne by people of color as well as low-income and rural populations in the United States (M. Good et al., 2005; Smedley et al., 2003; U.S. Department of Health and Human Services, 2001). In the context of poverty and homelessness, there is the added danger of medicalizing social and structural inequalities.

Within medicine and psychiatry, there is also recognition of the limitations of traditional biomedical approaches. More than 40 years ago, psychiatrist George Engel (1977) argued for "the need for a new medical model" (p. 129) in proposing the biopsychosocial approach. In making the case for psychiatry to embrace a broader definition of the nature and scope of problems within its purview, Engel (1977) links this to the ethical orientation and professional responsibility of the discipline: "The importance of how physicians conceptualize disease derives from how such concepts determine what are considered the proper boundaries of professional responsibility and how they influence attitudes toward and behaviors with patients" (p. 129). More contemporary efforts within medicine to move beyond narrow biomedical models include greater attention to social determinants of health (Braveman & Gottlieb, 2014) and calls for "structural competency" (Metzl & Hansen, 2014). Within mental health services, community-based models of care such as assertive community treatment (ACT) (Stein & Santos, 1998) as well as mobile outreach and "street psychiatry" are treatment approaches that strive to address mental health needs amid complex social and structural inequities.[1] Yet such services are often constrained by limited resources, and many front-line providers do not have the training or experience to meaningfully engage with the complex intersection of mental health and social needs (Brodwin, 2013). Moreover, as Helena Hansen and her colleagues (2018) have argued, the education of mental health professionals has not emphasized social determinants of mental health. Specific to homelessness, only half of psychiatry residency programs offer clinical rotations that include experience with homelessness, and only 20% of residents participate in the programs that do exist (McQuistion et al., 2004). Such constraints can produce gaps between the goals or intentions of care and the practical reality of services for people marginalized by mental health, substance use, and poverty.

In exploring the complex and often ineffective intersection between marginalized families and care providers, this chapter begins by detailing three patterns of paradoxes of care—on my terms, going through the motions, and grasping at straws. *On my terms* describes those who harbor skepticism toward institutions of care, maintain distance from health and social services, and are strongly oriented toward self-reliance. *Going through the motions* refers to those who participate in care but remain deeply ambivalent about aspects of therapeutic and supportive services. Finally, *grasping at straws* describes those who are heavily involved with a range of health and social service providers but do not experience significant changes within the areas of their lives that matter most. These three patterns underscore that there is not a singular trajectory in how marginalized families interact with service providers or navigate through systems of care. The patterns that I describe using emblematic examples grounded in the lived experiences of families can be understood as constituting a spectrum of orientations toward care. To more fully contextualize these individual experiences, I layer in the voices of a broader group of people with whom I engaged at Safe Harbor and also include perspectives from health and social service providers within the chapter. Following the discussion of paradoxes of care, I consider the impact of the ubiquity of services in the lives of many families, arguing that forms of help and support may be recast as modes of surveillance with unintended—and sometimes dire—consequences for marginalized families.

On My Terms: Critical Perspectives on Care

Over the years, Barbara and I had settled into an easy routine of running errands together and chatting over coffee at Dunkin' Donuts. Barbara was in her mid-40s and White and lived with her long-term partner, Evan, and her teenage children. An early riser by habit, Barbara always kept an eye out for my car, bustling out to greet me with a warm, "Well, hello, Elizabeth. So nice to see you." Quickly, I would be enveloped in her presence, the space between us blooming with the fragrance of her perfume, her signature painted nails, and her warm, lilting voice. Ever the news hound, Barbara would rush to tell me about the latest current events or her opinions on politics, her voice rising and falling by turns in astonishment, admiration, or indignation.

Barbara brought the same critical edge to her view of the medical establishment: "They put a label on everybody these days. . . . Our society is, like, 'If you take this, you'll be this. You won't have heart attacks anymore. Your blood pressure will go down.' Give me a break. I don't need any of that, and that's the way I feel." She was deeply skeptical of what she viewed as the proliferation of mental health and substance use diagnoses in the region. While Barbara was facile with clinical language and diagnostic categories, she largely eschewed "psy-" understandings, and, in her view, psychiatric medications were a distraction from the "root cause" of such problems:

> You're not dealing with the problem. You're just masking it. And you're just walking around in a cloud. You have no thought or no feeling. And nothing really bothers you because you're just numb to things. And that's why I don't think that all that medicine—I don't think it's good for people. I really don't. I think that people are convinced that it's magic in this bottle, and it's not. It's not. And over a period of time, I don't think that they've been able to rectify or help the problem that it just kind of gets worse. You're just kind of coddling it and, you know, giving it a little Band-Aid here and a Band-Aid there, when, you know, really are you at the problem?

Just as Barbara had criticized other parents at the shelter for "wanting things handed to them" (see chapter 2), she expected that people should strive to take care of problems on their own. Elaborating on her concerns about medications, Barbara emphasized the need for personal responsibility in dealing with mental illness and substance use:

> I don't wanna go see a therapist and have her give me all these medications. I'm sure with my story she would, too. I don't want you to douse me with medications. I want a clear head. If I'm not happy when I wake up in the morning, what do I need to change? . . . I'm sorry, but I think they try to shove it down our throats, and I think it's ridiculous especially with mental health. I mean, there isn't a medication out there that I haven't been on at one point or another, and none of it works until you change your ways.

Barbara's skepticism toward psychiatric care and her orientation to personal responsibility shaped how she responded to her own experiences with childhood trauma, depression, and substance use. In the past, she had engaged with mental health counseling and had been prescribed psychiatric medication. She described feeling "insulted by the counselor" at the community mental health center and had been frustrated that she was given "a ton of meds." Thinking back to this time, Barbara remembered the amber pill bottles that had lined her windowsill. Over time, she became increasingly disillusioned by "pharmaceutical promises" (Carpenter-Song, 2009b, p. 273): "I've been medicated before many times so I already know about all of that. And none of it did any good—any good at all. If anything, it made it kind of worse. . . . I mean, we're born into this world with nothing. I don't think we need anything to throw into our bodies like that." She recalled her decision to throw away her psychiatric medications. When she told her psychiatrist that she had thrown away all of her medications, the provider "yelled at me," leaving her feeling "humiliated." Still, Barbara remained steadfast and had told the psychiatrist: "I don't want to take all these meds!"

By the time we met, Barbara had completely disengaged from mental health services. Barbara also had not sought professional help for the serious substance use problem that had precipitated her family's homelessness (see chapter 2). Looking back on this difficult time, Barbara attributed her ability to stop using drugs to her own willingness to change, the support of her partner, and her religious faith:

> You've got to want it. And you know, I've had [partner] at my side, and we've done a great job with it. It's not something that a lot of people even know because I don't tell people. I don't brag on it—on how long it's been or anything else like that. I just know what my life was, and I know where I was at, and I was pretty bad. . . . You know, I lost everything I had, so I already know that feeling, what that's like. And the only thing that is going to help you is God. . . . People can do it. And there was no counselor. There was nothing. Nothing. Nothing. But him and I believing in each other and believing that God will take care of it. We'll be all right. We'll make it.

Barbara's own profound struggles complicate a more simplistic interpretation of her experience as constituting a hardline moralistic viewpoint. Hers is not an arm's-length critique of "others" but rather a perspective forged in the crucible of lived experience and the high stakes of stopping her drug use. For Barbara, keeping a distance from mental health and substance use services animated her daily efforts to sustain long-term sobriety and her mental health. Barbara's experience resonates with the "moral agency" embedded in U.S. recovery discourses described by Neely Myers (2015) and aligns strongly with the bootstrap mentality within rural New England. Crucially, Barbara's orientation toward self-reliance is more than a discursive framing of her experience. Her orientation has been linked to practical action that has made a difference for her family. She has learned to rely on herself and has maintained not only her sobriety and mental health but also her housing, despite cycling through low-paid service-sector jobs, the specter of debt, and the continued fragility of her family's financial situation. She is embedded in social services (such as subsidized housing) but engages with these services "on her own terms." As she stated early in the study in anticipation of moving out of Safe Harbor:

> When I leave, my feet will never set foot in these doors again. They won't. They won't. No. Nope nope, no. Because I went for thirty—thirty-five—years where, you know, I made it. I made it without any kind of service like that. You know, I didn't go pick up bread, I didn't go and have this. I made it. If I didn't have it, I didn't have it, and that was that. And that's the way I look at it. I won't go down and take. They have a thing where you can go and get food at the end of the month. I won't do that. Somebody else needs it more than me. I'll just go without.

She has deep faith in God and also herself: "Through my mind, I can get beyond whatever is bothering me. Out of this funk or whatever."

Going through the Motions: Ambivalent Engagement in Care

Unlike Barbara's rejection of mental health and substance use services, other families willingly participated in a variety of forms of care. Tara was in her mid-20s and White. She was raising a toddler son when we met and later had a daughter. Her relationship with her husband was fraught, with frequent break-ups and reunions. As I learned later, Tara experienced domestic violence. Tara had a long history of drug use. She first took opiates with her father as a teenager. Tara's interactive style was welcoming and friendly. When I visited, she asked after me and remembered details that I had shared with her. Often, we would talk at her small kitchen table, with the scent of a just-mopped floor wafting around us.

Tara traveled 90 minutes round-trip on a daily basis to a methadone clinic to treat her opiate addiction. She had been engaging in this daily effort for over five years. While she was hopeful that her treatment might end soon, the trajectory of her care was unclear: "I've been going down on my dose. Hopefully, that'll be done soon. It's been five years. It takes forever. It's taking me forever." Tara's willingness to go along with the inconvenience and serious disruption of time-consuming daily methadone treatments underscores her desire to move beyond her substance use ("I'm trying to do better") but also belies the ambivalence she held toward clinical services. During one of our conversations, Tara told me that her case worker "keeps trying to push this counseling thing on me. She really wants me to go see a counselor." I could sense an openness in her tone and said, "Well, you were thinking about it before." She sighed, seeming to weigh the possibility: "Yeah, I just don't know. It's kind of weird talking to somebody that I don't know about my fucked-up life."

A perceived lack of shared experience with clinical providers was also a reason that Nancy felt uncomfortable with the prospect of seeing a therapist for her depression, anxiety, and ADHD. Nancy was in her late 20s and White and was raising two children. With her wry sense of humor, Nancy did not hesitate to share her opinions. Early in the study, shortly after Nancy had moved out of Safe Harbor to double up with friends, I sat with Nancy and her housemate, Cindy, as the conversation turned to the struggles they had faced in their lives:

Cindy: I've dealt with everything: abusive relationships, abusive parents. Nancy's gone through the same stuff.

ECS: Have you guys ever talked to anybody about these things? Or not really?

Nancy: Like a therapist? No, it's all about the money with a therapist.

ECS: Really?

Nancy: Yeah, and they haven't been through the same things, so it doesn't help. They can say, "I understand," but they really don't.

I took Nancy's comment "it's all about the money with a therapist" to signal the perceived gulf between middle-class clinical providers and the experiences of those on the economic margins. This economic divide may amplify the sense that providers do not share similar backgrounds or life experiences, as Nancy questions the authenticity of claims by therapists that they "understand." In addition to social class, a perceived lack of shared experience with trauma may also widen the expected gap with care providers.

Nancy readily accepted the psychiatric diagnoses she had received over the years and was prescribed antidepressant and anti-anxiety medications for these conditions. She linked her worsening anxiety to living in a rural environment, describing the impact of isolation when she and her two small children moved to a remote Vermont town to access more affordable housing: "I didn't have this problem before I moved to [remote Vermont town]. My anxiety was not this bad. . . . And I think it was just being by myself with the kids for so long that it—I mean, I've always had the anxiety, but I just think it triggered it worse."

While she recognized that some people may benefit from therapy, "I choose personally not to do therapy right now because of—I hate therapy [laughs]." This was something that I had heard repeatedly from Nancy over the years, and I asked her to elaborate. She explained that she had been "doing therapy since I was—what? Six, seven years old" because of a custody issue with her birth father when her mother remarried. Later, as an adolescent, Nancy was sent to a therapist "because of the cutting and depression and the anger and everything." As a teen, Nancy had been placed in foster care when her behavior became too difficult for her family to manage. She continued:

> And then over the years as an adult, I've gone [to therapy], but I just get really frustrated 'cause therapists seem like they know it all. Or that you're making up excuses or cop outs. They just—I don't know. It's like they don't believe you or something like that. . . . It just seems like a lot of judgment and everything 'cause, you know, I know I've gotten myself into situations I shouldn't have, you know? But I'll own up to my mistakes, but it just seems like—I don't know. I don't know [laughs].

Rather than experiencing therapists as a supportive presence, Nancy highlighted her sense of feeling judged for certain actions or decisions in her life. Like Barbara, Nancy's critique was not a view from afar but rather a perspective drawn from a lifetime of engagement with social and mental health services.

During a period of time when Nancy moved to a southern state with the hope of accessing more affordable housing, she had her first positive experience with a mental health counselor. At one point after she returned to Vermont, I asked her to reflect on what was different about this experience:

> It didn't seem like therapy 'cause we would go shopping and stuff or just go—I still had [my son] at home 'cause we had moved into a shelter, and their pre-K was full in that town so he couldn't go. So while [my daughter] was at school,

we'd do stuff. One day, we took him to the fire station. You know what I mean? It was like a friendship almost. We'd just shoot the shit like you and I do. You know? And it was nice.

To elaborate on this positive experience, we continued our dialogue:

ECS: What could therapists do to improve what they're doing? I think a lot of people get into that field, and they wanna—they're trying to do the right thing, I think.

Nancy: They could have a more relaxed center and everything. Even if it's just the office. Make it so it doesn't look like an office almost? You know? Or do stuff like even just going for walks and talking. Just make it easier for people to talk. You know that's why it takes people so long to come out with stuff. I think [it] is 'cause the environment that they're in and the setting and everything. So that's what's always been my issue. I feel like if I'm going to a therapist's office, I'm going to the doctors. And I really hate doctors. So I only go once a year unless something is really wrong. That's why my hip hasn't been looked at yet.

ECS: What is it about doctors?

Nancy: I feel like I get judged there, too. And a lot of times—like, I'm afraid if I just go in for my hip, they'll tell me I need to lose weight. . . . I don't know. It just always comes around to that, and then that hits me emotionally 'cause, you know, I had an eating disorder in high school, so it's like, yeah, let's call somebody fat and tell them they have to lose weight who had an eating disorder! Luckily, I'm old enough and smart enough to know that's not healthy, and I won't go back to that, but, you know, it's still a constant reminder in the back of my head. The same thing when I get really depressed, the cutting's been back in my head, but I won't do it. That's also why I tattooed the kids' names on my wrist. To be a reminder, you know. But it's just—I'm strong enough to know better, but there are people out there that aren't.

Nancy's positive experiences with mental health services illuminate that her orientation to care is not ossified and point to specific features of therapeutic environments and interactions that aligned with her needs and expectations. Moreover, she speaks to how negative experiences in care become a shadow over future encounters and how expectations of judgment made her less likely to seek help.

Grasping at Straws: Intensive Engagement in Care

Jim and Hannah were a married couple in their 40s and the parents of four young children. They relocated to Vermont following an accident that left Jim disabled and moved with the hope of accessing better healthcare for their family. Jim and Hannah were deeply reflective in sharing their own experiences of housing insecurity and mental health challenges. They often placed these vulnerabilities in relation to their observations of social or systemic issues.

The couple stood out among the families for their strong alignment with clinical understandings and eager participation in a range of professional services as they contended with chronic physical and mental illnesses. Both readily accepted mental health diagnoses of depression, anxiety, and PTSD and viewed medication and psychotherapy as valuable modes of treatment. Jim and Hannah had long histories of involvement with mental health services and, unlike the ambivalence expressed by Tara and Nancy, actively sought out and valued the perspectives of mental health counselors. Hannah explained her perspective on the importance of access to mental health services, especially for those facing the challenges of poverty and housing insecurity:

> I think it is so imperative to have counseling, to have a mentor, to have an advocate, to have a counselor—somebody that you can sit with one moment during your week and go, "This is what's really going on. Help me sort this out." That's so imperative because if one was to have that in the very beginning, I could not imagine how different life would be for so many families.

As she continued, Hannah noted that it can be challenging to see the value in mental health services when people are focused on day-to-day survival:

> I had so much going on I felt like I didn't have time or the money [to see a therapist]. You're worrying about gas money, to go see a counselor or a therapist when you don't have heat. You know, you don't have [fire]wood. I mean it seems kinda senseless: why would I do that? That's on the last of the list. And I did that for a really long time until I just felt absolutely pushed into—I was really gonna succumb with complete depression and anxiety.

This sentiment was echoed by case managers at Safe Harbor who described how "the tyranny of the moment"—the daily focus on survival—could compromise the inherently longer-range vision involved in seeking mental health care.

Unlike Nancy's feelings of judgment from therapists, Jim and Hannah had strong connections to their therapists and trusted their perspectives. Jim would often share bits of advice or things that he had learned from his therapist. From Jim's accounts, his therapist validated the difficulties of his experiences and normalized his responses. During this time, Jim and Hannah were in a protracted custody process with the state of Vermont following the removal of their children nearly a year before (see chapter 5). When Jim began having vivid and sometimes violent dreams, his therapist said that Jim's feelings of anger were "normal" and that "I should be angry at everyone involved in this case." Although they deeply valued the affirmation and support they received from their therapists, there was also a practical limit to what these professionals were able to do in relation to improving the material conditions of life for this couple or for reuniting them with their children. To address these needs, Jim and Hannah turned to professionals in a range of other agencies and services.

Whereas they valued their interactions with their therapists, Jim and Hannah raised questions about the usefulness of their involvement with other professionals. One evening, as snow fell in fat flakes outside, I asked them to detail the professional services in which they were currently engaged. What I had thought was a simple question launched us into a conversation that stretched for hours as they described days and weeks consumed by appointments—with healthcare providers, vocational rehabilitation specialists, lawyers, child welfare workers, and housing services—as they made efforts to fulfill the court mandates to be reunified with their children:

Hannah: How many times I have spent *days* on the phone? I mean, the phone battery dies because you're trying to find a resource for this, a resource for that. And you can't get anywhere.

Jim: And then you add up all the agencies that we're involved with, we gotta meet with all of 'em at some point in time.

Hannah: And they *drain* us . . . all these visits with all these quote-unquote support people that stress me out, use my time, exhaust me. I don't get anything out of it. But I'm exhausted, really. My life is more invaded, and I'm not heard.

This exchange highlighted how, for this family, involvement with professional services had overshadowed their everyday lives. During this time, the couple did not have a car and spent hours on foot walking to attend appointments with service providers.

Despite their personal sacrifices and the numerous professionals with whom they interacted regularly, the couple continued to experience profound financial precarity and ongoing threats to their housing stability; intensifying substance use; and fundamental shifts in their sense of identity and purpose as they endured the continued separation from their children as will be detailed in chapter 5. Crucially, *more* services did not yield tangible benefits from the perspective of Jim and Hannah. Rather than a salve for the wounds of their loss, the intense involvement of professionals in their lives brought a sense of intrusion, as Hannah elaborated: "You feel really exposed. You wanna close in, wrap around tight around your family. You're focusing so much on that survival. You don't want more people involved. It's not that you don't want help, it's—You want some semblance of normalcy. You want some semblance of privacy." This sense of exposure and loss of privacy echoes Donna Friedman's (2000) argument that families experiencing homelessness "parent in public." The hallmark features of homelessness— poverty and displacement—render parents exquisitely vulnerable to the "gaze" of social workers, health professionals, law enforcement, and other "helping professions."

Family Portrait: A Home Visit and the Magnification of Daily Life

With the frame of "parenting in public" (Friedman, 2000), I turn now to consider the ubiquity of services in the lives of many families. Various "workers" were a regular presence in the lives of families. It was common to have case managers drop by to visit with parents and young children in their homes. Parents in the study understood that their access to resources— SNAP and TANF benefits, vouchers for school supplies and used furniture, occasional bags of diapers and cans of formula—was predicated on their cooperation with regular intrusions into the intimate spaces of domestic life. Just as in the shelter setting, some families found themselves under the watchful eye of case managers even after they had moved into their own homes. Such visits were usually anticipated nervously.

When I arrived at Nancy's apartment one afternoon, I found her fretting over the dishes piled in the sink and the trash bags that had collected in the kitchen. "I've gotta take those down to the dumpster before she [the case worker] comes." There was a knock at the door, and Nancy yelled out, "It's open." Katie, a case manager, stepped into the apartment and looked surprised to see me there. We smiled politely at one another. "This is Elizabeth. We're doing research," Nancy stated by way of explanation and introduction. Katie, who looked to be in her mid-20s, did not inquire further, and I did not elaborate on my role, leaving it to families to decide whether and how to describe our relationship to others. Dressed neatly in jeans and a red top, Katie greeted the children in a sing-song, high-pitched voice. Her eyes darted around the room as she looked for a place to sit, finally settling into a child-size purple papasan chair.

The focus of Katie's visit was a "session" with Nancy's daughter, Emily, who was three at the time. Nancy was expected to track when Emily performed certain activities—sharing, eating at the table, listening—by marking a behavioral chart with stickers. When Katie asked about the chart, Nancy pointed to the top of a cluttered dresser: "It's up there somewhere. When that's cleared off, maybe we'll start using that again." Katie nodded, "Okay, I'll just keep printing these out in the meantime." Katie turned her attention to going over what Emily had done well over the past week, doing her best to interest the preschooler in a packet of stickers. At one point, Emily picked up a bag of chips from the coffee table, reaching her small hand inside before brandishing the bright orange triangle. Katie seized the opportunity: "Emily, do you remember where you're supposed to be eating?" Still holding the chip, Emily blinked her large brown eyes and mumbled, "At the table." "That's right!" Katie exclaimed. "Do you think you can sit at the table?" Emily nodded and sat down at the table.

The session continued like this, with Katie prompting Emily to do certain things to earn stickers with the goal of earning a prize. During this particular session, it was the promise of a small mermaid toy. At one point, Katie shifted to a directed activity and played a game of Simon Says with Emily. At first, Emily was engaged, giggling at the directions, "Simon says: 'Touch your ear,'" "Simon says: 'Touch your knee,'" "Touch your nose.'" But as the game stretched on, Emily's attention drifted, and she grew increasingly boisterous, no longer following the prompts of the game. As Emily spun around and laughed loudly, Katie reminded her of the possibility of earning a prize. Instead of having the intended effect of refocusing attention to the game, Emily instead became fixated on getting the prize *now*. Katie wearily explained, "If you don't do what you need to do to earn the stickers, you won't get the mermaid," as Emily whined, "*Mer-maid*."

The session came to a close when Nancy's neighbor stopped by. Seemingly eager for the session to end, Katie ultimately gave Emily the required number of stickers for the mermaid prize before packing up her bag to leave.

This brief portrait of a home visit illustrates the blurring of boundaries between domestic and professional settings. For Nancy, quotidian dimensions of life became magnified through the lens of her "worker." Dirty dishes, unfolded laundry overflowing from a hamper, and crowded and cluttered rooms became signifiers of (in)stability—potential evidence of one's "fitness" as a parent. I thought of the gulf between the visibility of families like Nancy's and the privacy of my own as I observed the worker's scan of the apartment. In my mind's eye, I saw my own unwashed dishes in the kitchen sink, papers piled on the table, and the basket of laundry waiting to be folded. I wondered how the worker would see such disorder in my home environment: would I catch the same subtle judgment I had just seen flash across her young face? By engaging with various organizations to gain access to needed resources, families in the study risked having their financial and housing insecurity call into question their adequacy as parents. For the families in the study, "Their parenting is more visible to government and public agencies that that of their middle class counterparts" (Appell, 1998, p. 356). For some families, this visibility had the tragic consequence of fundamentally refashioning supportive services into an apparatus of surveillance and harm, as is elaborated in chapter 5, which details the gradual unraveling of life for two families in the wake of losing custody of their children.

Paradoxes of Care

In exploring the complex interface between marginalized families and care providers, this chapter focuses on the diverse orientations to biomedical, psychiatric, and social services found among families. This underscores the crucial contribution of attending closely to subjective experience in the context of mental health (Jenkins & Barrett, 2004) and also the need for specificity in considerations of marginalized families. Though these families shared many common experiences of economic precarity alongside forms of suffering diagnosable as mental health conditions, they varied considerably in their orientations toward professional services and preferred modes of engagement. This resonates with previous research showing that bionarratives are but one way that families come to understand and respond to suffering (Carpenter-Song, 2009a).

For Barbara, despite a history of childhood trauma and serious substance use, biomedical and "psy-" conceptualizations held little relevance. She instead held tightly to self-reliance and religious faith to make sense of these experiences and to inform her daily efforts that have enabled her sobriety and housing stability amid her family's fragile economic circumstances. Others, like Tara and Nancy, willingly participated in some aspects of mental health and substance use treatment but largely viewed professionals as out of touch with the harsh realities of living in poverty. Both described hesitancies engaging with middle-class clinicians who "haven't been through the same stuff." By contrast, Jim and Hannah found psychiatric renderings of suffering to be useful and actively sought mental health services. They were heavily involved with a range of professionals in organizations spanning mental health, housing, child welfare, and the legal system. Interacting with these service providers required vast amounts of time and personal sacrifice by Jim and Hannah. Yet their substantial efforts to interface with professional services appeared to do little to catalyze meaningful change toward stability or the reunification of their family. Fragmented services left these parents exhausted and critical of systems.

The diverse orientations to mental health challenges, treatment, and services that I found among families in the study were also manifest in others with whom I interacted at Safe Harbor over the years. Some spoke to the difficulties of living with the multiple burdens of mental illness and poverty, as Linda commented:

> It's a challenge when you live with mental health issues. It's a challenge getting through every day. It's a challenge accessing services. It's a challenge with trying medications. It's a challenge with staying on your medications. It's a challenge with having the financial resources to pay for the copayments.

Others at Safe Harbor drew connections between their mental health and substance use and aspects of living in a rural setting. James described how his drinking escalated when he was living in a remote area: "I was drinking heavily—um, three to four bottles of wine a day. Because I was isolated. The nearest house was a mile away. I mean, it was totally in the wilderness. And so I decided to go to a hospital, psychiatric hospital, because I was worried I was going to hurt myself, very depressed."

Some noted that the lack of anonymity in small, rural towns made them reluctant to seek treatment. Kimberly described the stigma that can accompany having mental health problems in rural environments:

> The worst thing is that everybody knows that you have any issues. The whole town knows. That is not always a good thing. Especially in certain small towns around here, there's a lot of people with an old-school way of thinking. If you have a mental illness or anything, then there's something wrong with you. That means you're not going to work in that town. You're not going to be looked at the same. You know? I worked at a little general store for nine years. Just the gossip that goes through there about people that have issues, I've watched it ruin so many people's lives in that town. Nobody even realizes they're doing it by telling one person and then that person happens to tell somebody who's against this. I think that's really the hard part with the small town.

In a setting in which self-reliance forms a prominent ethos, others at Safe Harbor described "a pride thing" and the sense that "I can handle it" as limiting their willingness to seek help. Many also echoed the sentiments of skepticism, mistrust, and disappointment that shadowed the lives of Barbara, Tara, Nancy, Jim, and Hannah. Among those struggling with substance use, judgment and stigma within healthcare encounters were commonly described. Eric shared his negative experiences with seeking care: "So the stigma thing is a huge deal. And doctors are absolutely disgusting when it comes to that. I bet I've seen over a hundred [doctors] and probably two were kind. There's no kindness. They roll their eyes and say, 'What do you want to do now?,' you know?"

Interviews with a broader range of Safe Harbor participants revealed strong critiques of the perceived overuse of psychotropic medications. Ben described negative subjective effects of medications and expressed his desire to take care of problems on his own: "Medication sometimes doesn't even help it. It makes me feel like I'm drugged up when I'm on medication. I don't want to be taking medication at all. I really don't. I'd rather deal with it the way I know how to do it." As Ben continued, he described experiencing childhood trauma and several injuries that had left his "brain fried." In his view, mental health professionals "think medication is going to take care of it, but it doesn't. It just covers it up is what it does." Speaking to the limitations of medication-focused treatments, Donna put the issue within a broader context of state-funded healthcare that limits options to diverse forms of treatment:

> There's not a lot of help for mental health, I find, as you find more help with drug abuse help. At least from the area that I came from, I found it was very difficult [to access mental healthcare], unless you had the right insurance or something. Nobody would really help you and all the doctors wanted to do was push pills down your throat. They didn't want to find a natural way of resolving issues. I didn't want to rely on medication to resolve it. There definitely needs to be more accessibility to get other help than just a pill that the state will cover.

Ben also expressed his wish for other forms of care beyond medication: "Not being in a hospital. Not being in a room where you have to be poked and prodded and drugged up all the time. You don't need it. All you need is someone to hug and listen to you and sit there. A nice counselor would be nice. That you can actually trust."

These perspectives on health and social services reflected long histories of needs that were not met, clinical encounters that were heavy with stigma, and limited options to pursue a range of therapeutic modalities.

I believe that at least part of the reason for the misalignment observed between marginalized populations and care providers in rural New England is rooted in the lack of attention to matters of social class in this context and indeed, more broadly, in the United States (Ortner, 1998). When class differences are acknowledged but not linked in informed ways to forms of structural inequality (Metzl & Hansen, 2014), there is the risk that care providers will misapprehend forms of suffering as "merely" individual pathology rather than as complex, reciprocal modes of struggle that link psychiatric symptoms to institutional structures of power (Jenkins, 2015b; Jenkins & Csordas, 2020). The experiences of the families and others at Safe Harbor compel consideration of reasons for the tenuous or haphazard engagement of rural populations in mental health and substance use services. Phrases such as "lack of engagement" or "noncompliance" gloss deeper realities of the harms that may be experienced by those marginalized by mental illness, substance use, and poverty in the context of professional services. As Kim Hopper (2006) has argued: "When deprivation is reckoned in the dual registers of material want and moral worth, the price of relief is paid in the currency of self-regard. Under such circumstances, what looks like a rejection of service or assistance may actually be a refusal to pay the toll" (p. 219). Attending closely to lived experience illuminates how differences in social class between patients and providers create conditions that cultivate skepticism and mistrust; how past experiences of feeling "judged" cast a long shadow over future engagement with care providers; how the New England bootstrap mentality, with its expectations of self-reliance, and pervasive stigma in small, rural towns may discourage help seeking; and how engaging in services may be experienced as intrusive, transforming help into unwelcome and potentially harmful forms of surveillance.

Following families as they navigated through the landscape of care in rural New England has highlighted rifts in their experiences of engaging with the systems intended to support them. These points of disconnect contribute to the paradoxes of care observed as families struggling with chronic health, mental health, and substance use challenges in the context of poverty remained tenuously and haphazardly engaged with professional services. In some cases, these slippages arose from divergent explanatory models (Kleinman, 1980) of the nature of suffering. Barbara offers an example of such misalignment in her strong rejection of clinical understandings and treatment. Some individuals will prefer to remain outside of professional mental health and substance use services, finding meaningful support instead through family, community, or faith. Reframing the rejection of services as a form of strength may create opportunities to bridge the seeming divide between individuals like Barbara and systems of care during periods of intense suffering.

In other cases, these slippages represent missed opportunities to engage families more meaningfully in supportive services. In rural areas, missed opportunities may manifest because of limited access to mental health services (Thomas et al., 2009; Thomas et al., 2012). Care providers pointed to the importance of *support at the right time* as being critical to impactful care:

> It takes a lot of strength of character and a lot of motivation in order to get out of the situations that they've been in. I think if we can give the support and the consistency of support and if we hit it at the right time in somebody's life when they're open to wanting to take steps in improving their life and they've got a good backup, then I think we really can be effective. (Case manager, Safe Harbor)

Yet in rural settings with limited access to mental health services, critical windows of opportunity may be missed when someone is open to engaging with care providers but unable to make an appointment or begin treatment in a timely manner. Two social service providers described barriers to accessing mental healthcare in the Upper Valley:

> You can't find a psychiatrist anywhere right now—you can't get in to see a psychiatrist anywhere right now. It's a huge hole [in services].

> I haven't lived that long in the Upper Valley, but from what I gather, there is a shortage of mental health assistance, psychiatrists, and so forth. So it's very hard to get an appointment right away. I mean, the length of time before you can see somebody is difficult.

With specialty mental health services limited in rural settings, primary care often serves as the de facto mental health system (Fox et al., 1995) where medication-based treatment is the dominant mode of care (Jenkins & Snell-Rood, 2021). In addition, Medicaid limits the range of providers that people can see, as one shelter leader with mental health training explained:

> People who have Medicaid are limited in what providers they can see. Most private therapists—who are usually more experienced and skilled—do not accept Medicaid as a form of insurance, so people who are poor do not have access to those professionals. They often have already had negative experiences at their local community mental health centers and do not want to return there.

Many participants also critiqued the dominance of pharmacological approaches and voiced the importance of a range of therapeutic options.

Beyond the challenges of limited access to a full spectrum of mental health care in rural settings, mental health and social service providers also acknowledged the limitations of professional services in addressing the complex needs of families. Several staff members at Safe Harbor shared their perspectives on why their services may not align with families' views or priorities. As one shelter leader explained, when families first enter the shelter,

> they are so overwhelmed with their own needs and issues that they can't get out of their own way to take some steps that would be better for them . . . and sometimes we say that they're not ready, or we label it that they're not willing or not able to use services or whatever. The reality is that they're living in a place that somehow isn't connecting with the way that we think they could most quickly succeed. And so we're not relevant then to what's happening to them. . . . What we're saying doesn't feel sensible to them, so they don't follow through on things that are recommended or requested of them, and then that's hard.

This narrative reframes the perennial clinical problem of "noncompliance" through a lens of compassion. Although she acknowledged the difficulty of families not following through on recommendations, she offered a nuanced interpretation of how services may not be viewed as relevant in the context of the overwhelming experience of a housing crisis. This echoes

Hannah's observations that the relevance of mental health services may pale in comparison to more pressing survival needs. Relatedly, other care providers noted the importance of openness regarding the limits of treatment, as this shelter leader explained:

> I think sometimes people find therapy as not helpful due to their false expectations that therapy will "fix them." I think when they have therapy and it does not meet this expectation, then they have this notion that therapy is not helpful. It is important for therapists to educate clients on realistic expectations of therapy.

Her observation points to the importance of care providers being clear about the goals of treatment and acknowledging the very real limits of services to lessen the impact of structural forces of poverty.

Another shelter leader described the "constant challenge" of cultivating ongoing empathy among staff members:

> Something I've noticed that comes up a lot is when people first come into the shelter, many of them are just very depressed and upset about their situation, and they lose a lot of hope. They become hopeless. So they don't have a huge amount of motivation right off the bat to improve their situation, and at times staff can perceive people as being lazy or taking advantage of Safe Harbor and the services that we offer. So it takes constant effort and reminders for staff to help them maintain empathy for the situations that people are coming to us in. So that's a challenge, and it's a constant challenge.

Other staff members acknowledged the limitations of not sharing similar backgrounds or experiences with the shelter guests, as this case manager noted:

> It's all about trying to find a balance with their experience. Meeting them halfway. And, you know, they really resent especially being told what to do by people who have not been in their position. So I completely get that. And I have not been in their situation in terms of having lived in poverty or any kind of drug history, you know?

Commenting on the differences in the lived experiences between middle-class care providers and people living in poverty, a community psychiatrist noted that many of the people he has worked with over the years have experienced significant trauma alongside few stable and trusting relationships in their lives. Working with patients, he endeavors to begin from a perspective in which skepticism and expectations of mistrust are not only to be expected but are understood as useful adaptations within a life marked by suffering and precarity. Elaborating on his therapeutic approach, he shared things that he has tried to teach psychiatric residents and case managers:

Don't try to *help*. Try to *understand* what this individual is experiencing. Try to understand how the individual has developed his or her personality and relationships based on a life of experiences. Diagnosis is trivial, especially in comparison to context. Medical solutions for social problems are expensive and ineffective. Who does this individual trust to help? It's rarely a doctor or social worker. How does he or she learn? It's unlikely to be from professional advice.

Missed Opportunities

The conceptual frame of missed opportunities begins from the foundational assumption that most health and social service providers are well intentioned in their work. While this may seem like a statement of the obvious, traditional critiques of biomedicine elide the "moral impulse" at the heart of medical practice (cf. B. Good, 1994) and, as such, do not provide an adequate basis for theorizing the misalignment between motives and practice. As Byron Good (1994) has noted: "One could read Foucault's description of the hospital and medical practice, as well as much medical anthropology, with little sense of the moral and soteriological core of experience that is present" (p. 86).

By contrast, the meaning-centered and experience-based orientation (Kleinman, 1988; B. Good, 1994; Jenkins, 2015a) of this research offers points of entry for engaging with the tensions experienced by providers as they struggle to provide compassionate care within the constraints of contemporary medical and social services. Scholarship conducted with this orientation has foregrounded biomedicine as a moral enterprise (B. Good, 1994) as providers negotiate between "competence and caring" (M. Good, 1995). More specific to the experiences of marginalized families, previous research has shown how bureaucratic organizational demands and policy structures detract from clinicians' efforts to engage meaningfully with patients with complex mental health and social needs (Brodwin, 2013; Bullon et al., 2011; Lipsky, 2010). This body of work underscores that a critical perspective alone is inadequate to the task of engaging with complex landscapes of care and offers opportunities for reimagining possibilities for meaningful supports for individuals, families, and communities (cf. Whitley, 2014). This perspective recasts the work of providers as a form of moral striving (Mattingly, 2014)—well-intentioned, imperfect efforts to care in the context of constraints.

Yet it is also the case that a "moral impulse" alone is insufficient protection against the forces of socialization that erode empathy and amplify cynicism in medicine (Hojat et al., 2004); the incremental assaults of long hours, inadequate supports, and low pay in social services (Mor Barak et al., 2001); and systemic racism and institutional bias in healthcare (M. Good et al., 2005; Hansen, 2019; Smedley et al., 2003). The impress of these forces is evident among participants in the study in their experiences of feeling judged, their skepticism toward the motivations of providers, and the sense that providers are not attuned to "what really matters" (Kleinman, 2007). In the course of this work, these forces have shown through at times in dismissive reactions to the research. In one such instance, following a presentation at psychiatry grand rounds, a nurse in the audience commented: "*Those* women come in to have their babies, but then we *never see them again.*" The forces of cynicism were again apparent in the words of a psychiatry resident who challenged me during a seminar in which, after presenting my research, I prompted the group to consider the responsibilities of physicians in engaging with patients with mental health and complex social needs: "That's not why I went to medical school."

While there might be satisfaction in offering an incisive critique of such responses, this does little in practice to disrupt these unexamined assumptions and harmful power dynamics. Instead, I embed such commentary within the frame of missed opportunities to meaningfully support families in order to highlight the need for attention to conditions and structures that will more readily reconnect motivation to practice and create more fertile ground for the cultivation of "recognition" (Carpenter-Song, 2011) of marginalized families within systems of care. This interpretive stance opens a space to consider how students, trainees, and professionals come to narrow their view of the work of care and illuminates the shadows of unintended consequences of care. Crucially, the frame of missed opportunities asks what might be done to fan the embers of care providers' moral striving and to build capacities to examine systems and structures that produce harm in order to engage across difference with openness, curiosity, and a desire to learn from the complexity and messiness of patients' lived experiences.

The clarion call for a "new medical model" (Engel, 1977, p. 129) has yet to be fully realized, and the limits of traditional healthcare education and training opportunities continue to leave many providers lacking the knowledge and skills needed to meet the needs of individuals and communities marginalized by mental illness, addiction, poverty, racism, and stigma. Approaches that foreground the intersection of structural forces and health (Metzl & Hansen, 2014) and immerse providers with those experiencing homelessness (Lo et al., 2021) hold deep promise. In addition, as shelter leaders and mental health professionals in the study observed, many enter supportive services with few trusting relationships and histories of trauma. A narrow focus on symptoms, diagnosis, and pharmaceutical or psychotherapeutic treatment in the absence of attunement to the broader context of suffering will miss opportunities to build trust and, over time, pathways to healing. Health and social service providers need education and training in both trauma-informed approaches and social determinants of health to recognize the dual role of personal histories of violence and victimization (Harris & Fallot, 2001; Liu et al., 2021) and structural violence (Farmer, 1996) among people experiencing homelessness and living with mental health or substance use challenges. The diverse views on mental health services explored in this chapter illuminate the numerous ways resistance toward treatment may manifest. Reframing such resistance as both reasonable *and* as points of departure for therapeutic work—rather than impediments to it—may bend the arc of engagement toward trust, openness, and healing. In practical terms, this could involve orienting people to care as they enter services in order to collaboratively set expectations, acknowledge limits of therapeutic approaches, and openly discuss negative experiences with health and social service providers and demoralizing bureaucratic systems.

Individual health and social service providers bear responsibility for turning toward suffering and for cultivating conditions that will foster trust. Working across axes of difference and the multiple registers of stigma—poverty, mental illness, addiction—can be modeled on ethnographic modes of inquiry that apply open-ended questions to seek context and detail, strive to minimize power imbalances, and engage with curiosity and humility to learn from others (Carpenter-Song et al., 2007; Carpenter-Song, 2011). While some providers will take their responsibility further and engage in "committed work" that "goes beyond the call of duty" (Hopper, 2006 p. 221) to directly address the complex needs of people living on the margins, we cannot rely on the heroism of individuals. Put another way, we cannot leave the high stakes of respectful, equitable, and effective care to chance.

Providers need to be supported by institutional structures and policies that align the intentions of care with the realities of practice.

As we work collaboratively to meaningfully embed knowledge of the impress of systems and structures within the education and training of health and social service providers, the words of a psychiatrist colleague may be a useful point of departure for recentering the work of care. I am told he encourages all the residents in his department to see every encounter with a patient as an opportunity. These words link an orientation toward possibility and a valence of hope with a practical call to action. Framing the work of care in this way positions healthcare and social services as forms of advocacy and may, in turn, create conditions to acknowledge and begin to repair the wounds of social defeat (Luhrmann, 2007) in the service of health equity and social justice.

5 Shattered Families

In this chapter, I build on arguments presented in chapter 4 highlighting the challenges families in this study experienced while navigating complex systems of care in rural New England. This chapter elaborates on the frequent misalignment of the goals of health and social services and the lived reality of care by focusing on unintended consequences of the professional gaze. Specifically, this chapter traces the devastating subjective effects of losing children to state custody in the context of homelessness, mental illness, and substance use. Research on child welfare overwhelmingly focuses on child outcomes, and much less is known about the impact on parents of the involvement of child welfare professionals and the separations of families. Through ethnographic attention to the experiences of two families, I examine these traumatic separations to argue that a form of madness is produced at the nexus of state systems of power and that the rupture of intersubjective familial ties results in the gradual erosion and eventual loss of parental selves.

Homelessness as Moral Failure in Rural New England

As earlier chapters highlight, the lack of anonymity, intense individualism, and expectations of self-reliance in rural New England create conditions in which the loss of housing is frequently cast as a personal failure within one's social network. This view is also, tragically, often internalized by the displaced themselves. Becoming homeless in this setting renders families as morally suspect (cf. Hopper, 2003). Under these conditions, parents must actively demonstrate their "moral worthiness" (Snell-Rood and Carpenter-Song, 2018) through efforts to prove their "virtue" as good enough parents.

It is against this harsh backdrop that we must understand experiences of losing children to state custody in Vermont. Previous anthropological research on this topic has delineated how a cascade of crises—domestic violence, substance abuse, homelessness—eventuate in the separation of children from their mothers (Barrow & Lawinski, 2009). In Susan Barrow and Terese Lawinski's (2009) research among mothers experiencing homelessness and mental health and/or substance use challenges, most (71%) children went to live with extended kin in the context of family separations. In their sample of 61 families living in metropolitan New York State, most of whom were headed by women of color, family separations occurred largely outside of the child welfare system as "decisions about care were negotiated between parents and kin" (Barrow & Lawinski, 2009, p. 13). Informal, kinbased arrangements were "overwhelmingly preferred" over nonkin foster care by the mothers in the study, who "viewed child welfare agencies as capricious and punitive" (Barrow & Lawinski, 2009, pp. 13, 15). Barrow and Lawinski (2009) argue that separations of this kind point to the agency of disenfranchised mothers as they actively seek out respite for themselves or protection for their children; these strategies align with the sharing of resources and the responsibility of child-rearing documented among Black families in the seminal work of Carol Stack (1974).

The experiences of family separation that I examine in this chapter differ substantially from those documented by Barrow and Lawinski (2009). Most important, for the families I describe, their children were taken forcibly and unexpectedly into state custody. These separations were not acts of agentive parents striving to prevent or mitigate difficulties within their families by engaging kin networks to care for children. Rather, these separations were experienced as traumatic ruptures in the fabric of family life, involving the swift intervention of child welfare and law enforcement officials. As such, the family separations detailed in this chapter align closely with experiences described by legal scholar and activist, Dorothy Roberts (2021, 2022), who has documented the impact of the child welfare system within Black and low-income communities in the United States. Roberts (2021) describes the child welfare system as an "assemblage of public and private child protection agencies, foster care, and preventive services" that serve as a "crucial part of the carceral machinery" in marginalized communities (p. 67). Furthermore, Roberts (2022) argues that the "foundational logic" of the child welfare system, which she terms the family policing system, is "centered on threatening politically marginalized families with child removal" (p. 27).

While rates of child removal and termination of parental rights vary widely by state in the United States, Vermont consistently ranks among the top states for rates of child removal and the termination of parental rights (Bech, 2015). Compared to all other New England states and most of the nation, Vermont terminates the parental rights of children ages birth to three at a higher rate (Bech, 2015). In Vermont, termination of parental rights (TPR) petitions increased 60% between 2012 and 2016, mirroring a dramatic rise in abuse and neglect case filings over the same period (State of Vermont Judiciary, 2017). Increases in abuse and neglect cases and TPR petitions are largely attributed to the opioid crisis in Vermont (Walsh, 2016).

Neighboring New England states have also experienced increases in reports of child abuse and neglect, but states respond to these reports differently. For example, New Hampshire and Vermont have similar rates of children subject to an investigated report of abuse or neglect (43 and 42 per 1,000, respectively). Yet Vermont confirms maltreatment in 8 per 1,000 cases compared to 3 per 1,000 cases in New Hampshire (a rate 2.6 times higher) (Annie E. Casey Foundation, 2017). Out-of-home placements also differ between the states, with 4 per 1,000 children ages birth to 17 in foster care in New Hampshire compared to 11 per 1,000 in Vermont (Annie E. Casey Foundation, 2017). Such differences underscore the contested ground of child welfare involvement. Some argue that New Hampshire rates are too low, reflecting inadequate resources for the Department of Children and Families (Wallner, 2017). On the other hand, Matt Valerio, the Vermont defender general who oversees the court-appointed attorneys representing parents in TPR cases, acknowledged a shift toward removal of children in drug-related cases that previously may not have resulted in removal. Furthermore, he acknowledged the role of poverty in these cases: "To be perfectly frank, this isn't a legal problem at all. This is a poverty problem. A treatment problem, a housing problem, a jobs problem, all arising out of poverty" (Walsh, 2016). Furthermore, in the vast majority of TPR cases, the court rules in favor of the state such that, as reported by one local press article, "the state breaks up a Vermont family almost every day" (Walsh, 2016).

The Moral Threat of Parenting on the Margins: The Impact of Mental Illness and Poverty

Families surviving in poverty in rural New England face stigma and social rejection associated with not having the signifiers of the "good life" in the United States (see chapter 3). Moreover, lacking a stable home is often experienced as a personal failure in the context of the New England bootstrap culture, leading to intense shame and concern about what it means to be a "good parent" under conditions of economic precarity alongside mental health and substance use challenges. Custody decisions in the context of mental illness provide a site for empirical investigation at the intersection of state intervention, social policy, and mental health. Parents with mental illnesses are at high risk for the involvement of the child welfare system and the loss of child custody. While there remains limited data on this issue, some studies have reported custody loss rates as high as 75% (Mowbray, Oyserman, Zemencuk, & Ross, 1995). Experiencing an inpatient psychiatric episode (regardless of diagnosis) independently conferred a twofold higher risk of child welfare system involvement and a nearly threefold higher risk of having a child placed in out-of-home care (Park et al., 2006).

At a broader policy level, the federal Adoption and Safe Families Act (ASFA, Public Law 105-89) has implications for parents with mental illnesses. The ASFA was passed with bipartisan support to become law on November 19, 1997, and was designed to limit foster care drift and promote permanency in children's living situations. The ASFA mandated expedited timelines for permanency hearings and termination of parental rights proceedings. If a child has been in an out-of-home placement for 15 out of the past 22 months, the ASFA requires states to move to terminate parental rights to free children for adoption (ASFA, Public Law 105-89). Yet 15 months may be inadequate for parents with mental health or substance use problems to access and meaningfully engage with services, as Joanne Nicholson and colleagues (2001) note:

> While the intent of the ASFA is to protect the health and safety of children, the implementation of the law also seems, in many instances, to be detrimental to the interests of parents with mental illness . . . [and] may have unintended consequences in its implementation. The incentives for permanency planning may motivate child welfare agencies to focus on out-of-home placement and planning for children in the allotted timeframe, rather than to tackle the oftentimes complex needs of parents with mental illness. (p. 27)

The high risk of child welfare system involvement among parents with mental illness is compounded by the moral threat of parenting in poverty. Child welfare agencies are involved disproportionately in families with low incomes (Fong, 2017), and poverty is the most consistent characteristic among families with disabilities in which neglect is found (Kay, 2009). Although some research disputes class bias in the overrepresentation of poor children in the child welfare system (Jonson-Reid et al., 2009), other research supports reporting bias in finding that class and race are powerful predictors of whether an incident was reported to a child welfare agency (Hampton & Newberger, 1985). Black, Latinx, and Indigenous populations are overrepresented in the U.S. child welfare system (Roberts, 2022). Families with low incomes and those that have a parent with a disability become visible to health and social service agencies as they seek needed resources for their families, but they risk having poverty or mental illness call into question their capacities as parents (Appell, 1998; National Council on Disability, 2012).

For several reasons, in this chapter, I do not take a definitive stance regarding the rightness or wrongness of the legal decisions to involuntarily remove children in the specific cases described. I could make an appeal to ethnographic neutrality, although this admittedly feels thin when so much is at stake. In addition, I am not an expert on family law. My reservations are rooted in an ethical pragmatism that recognizes the limits of ethnographic knowledge and my understanding of these families. As an ethnographer, this work has entailed continuous negotiation of my ambiguous positionality. The immediacy of bearing witness to profound suffering exists in fraught tension with my commitment as an engaged scholar striving for impact. This has involved tempering appeals for direct advocacy by cultivating mutual understandings of the responsibilities and limits of our relationships.[1]

My ethnographic attention focuses on an emergent understanding of the devastating subjective effects of losing custody of children to the state. I have chosen to foreground the experiences of two families to underscore that these experiences are not singular. Presenting ethnographic material from two families also highlights distinctive contours, including an emphasis on drug use in Tara's case and mental illness in Jim and Hannah's experience. Through this work, I hope to raise critical questions about practices surrounding child separations, particularly in the context of homelessness and mental illness. Again, as Nicholson and her colleagues (2001) have written:

> Ultimately, the costs of severing family ties must be empirically documented and weighed against the benefits of out-of-home placement and permanency planning on a case-by-case basis for families in which parents have mental illness. Research is needed to evaluate the costs and benefits of one choice over the other. (p. 28)

Shattered Families, Loss of Parental Selves

Attention to the lived experience of family separations reveals crucial points of vulnerability and also of opportunity. Building on themes from the previous chapter, the experiences of Tara, Jim, and Hannah illuminate the high stakes involved in the misalignment of marginalized families and systems of care. In tracing the subjective effects of the removal of children and termination of parental rights by the state, I examine the consequences for parents as they endure profound loss and engage in ongoing efforts to be reunited with their children.

I use the vocabulary of *loss of self* to conceptualize the subjective effects of losing children to state custody.[2] The gradual unraveling of life for these two families in the wake of traumatic separations from their children threatens their identities and capacities as mothers and fathers striving to care for their children. Over time, some wounds cut so deep as to fundamentally alter self-processes to a point of devastation.[3] In the years following the removal of their children, Tara, Jim, and Hannah had their weaknesses amplified as the separations upended daily routines and rituals of caregiving that gave both structure and meaning to family life. Despite ongoing efforts to meet formal conditions of reunification, separations were prolonged, leaving these parents in a state of "existential limbo" (Haas, 2017) that incrementally eroded their capacities to care for their children. As the possibility that their children would return home receded, parental selves were lost amid the shattering of their families.

Family Portraits of Moral Striving and Loss

Tara was in her late 20s and White. She had a high school education and worked intermittently in service-sector jobs. She and her husband, Chris, had an on-again-off-again relationship. Tara had filed restraining orders against Chris at various points and later, filed for divorce. Tara reported having received psychiatric diagnoses including attention deficit disorder, bipolar disorder, and PTSD. When I met Tara in 2009 she had one toddler son and was working hard to maintain her sobriety after having started using opiates and other drugs as an adolescent. After spending nine months in the family shelter, Tara moved into a subsidized apartment in her hometown in

Vermont. She attributed her move to the support of the staff at Safe Harbor and also to her own persistence:

> I called on this apartment every single day. *Every single day.* I was persistent. I was very persistent. I did something for my son. I needed it. It's something that I needed to do, that I *had* to do. You know what I mean? I'm not just gonna sit back and relax. . . . Life is what you make it, and if you don't make it, you ain't gonna have one. [Another shelter resident] was outside crying the other day, "I'm gonna be here forever!" It's your own fault, you know? If I can do it, anybody can.

Tara was relieved to be out the shelter, where she had faced stigma from other residents for being in methadone treatment: "I'm in treatment. I get swabbed every week. If I used [drugs], I'd be screwed. So don't call me an addict." She enjoyed settling into her new apartment and felt that "people have been treating me different since I got a place. I just feel so much better about myself not being in the shelter anymore." Though sparsely decorated, she had taken care to place framed photographs on the bookshelf. The rooms were tidy and bright. Lacy sheer curtains hung delicately in her kitchen window. Shortly after Tara moved in, I complimented her on the apartment, and she beamed, "Oh, do you like it? I redecorated since you were here."

I looked forward to my visits with Tara. After picking up iced coffees from the Cumberland Farms convenience store, we would often drive to local thrift stores, where Tara would browse through the latest offerings. Along the way, we would talk about the things that were happening in her life. One afternoon, as we wound our way through town, she pointed to a small clapboard house: "That's where I grew up." She went on to share that her father had introduced her to heroin when she was in high school. Although she was grateful for her subsidized apartment, being in her hometown and near her family brought with it a map of memories—parking lots where she had bought drugs, houses where she had used—that made charting a new course a challenge from the start. During the time that I knew her, she oscillated between periods of sobriety and use.

When Tara first moved into the apartment, she was confident in her ability to pay the rent: "$198 a month, I'll be there forever. That's it, yeah. Yep, I can pay $198 dollars a month. And everything's included."[4] She articulated her sense that "things are coming together" and her desires for stability for her young family: "I mean, we are stable now with the apartment. I just want [my son] to be stable with me." As the months passed, Tara's narrative of stability shifted to one of loneliness and boredom: "It's been very lonely. There's nothing to do here. I just stay at home all day." At one point, Tara thanked me for coming over and added, "You're, like, my only friend." She elaborated her frustration with her neighbors, who "drink all day." Speaking about one of the women, Tara noted that "she wakes up and cracks open a beer. It's, like, I'm bored, but I'm not *that* bored." She shared her usual routine and her decision to start going to church:

Tara: Stressful. I sit at home every day, all day. It gets so old. I walk to [town] and back. And then I bring [my son] to the park. But other than that, I'm home 24/7.

ECS: Are you still writing in your journal?

Tara: Yes! Every day. Yeah, that's one thing I do. I write in my journal. I used to have more hobbies.

ECS: What about—do you think you'll meet anybody through church?

Tara: I don't know. I just started about four weeks ago. And I feel good! Like, when I go. You know? I mean, I'm not a huge churchgoer, you know what I mean? But it feels good to go, you know what I mean? Just to be associated with good people.

Living in her hometown, Tara continued to make efforts to meet new people but also struggled to distance herself from her old friends and family members, including her husband, with whom she maintained a complicated relationship. In the fall of 2010, about six months after moving into her apartment, she was pregnant with her second child. During this time, she had little support from her husband, the baby's father (see chapter 3). Still, Tara was eagerly anticipating the birth of her daughter. During our drives together, Tara would often thumb through her dog-eared copy of *What to Expect When You're Expecting*, sharing passages with me along the way. She worked for months to carefully decorate the nursery with serendipitous finds from secondhand stores. Her use of marijuana to soothe vicious morning sickness had been, if not officially sanctioned, tolerated by her healthcare providers. As she distanced herself from others, she was enjoying more time with her toddler-age son:

> He has been really, really good. I haven't been talking to people. I just exclude myself from people. I think that it is better. You know, it's just better to stay away from all of those people. So I have been spending more time with [my son]. And

we read at nighttime a lot. He is excited about coloring. And he seems calm. He hasn't been running back and forth like he usually does.

Yet Tara's trajectory of stability was again challenged a few months later. She relied on Medicaid-funded rides to transport her to her daily methadone treatment. After a driver complained that her son was "too loud" and "distracting" in the car, he was no longer allowed to join her on these 90-minute round-trip rides. Still needing to engage in daily treatment, Tara was left scrambling to find childcare. Her efforts to distance herself from her old friends and associates came to an abrupt halt as the immediate need for childcare for her young son took priority. She reengaged with an old family friend who arranged a babysitter. Initially, this friend provided much needed support, including pitching in for a used car. Yet, as I would learn in the coming months, reengaging with this friend also drew Tara back into her old networks and patterns of drug use.

"The state took my kids." Tara's words, delivered on my cell phone as I drove home from work one early summer evening, were urgent. Her anguish was palpable even at a distance. I was shocked. Just a month earlier, Tara had given birth to her daughter. Yet the newborn baby tested positive for drugs in the hospital, and this catalyzed Tara's involvement with child welfare officials. The involvement of the child welfare system escalated when Tara and a friend were arrested for drug possession, prompting the removal of her children by the state. In the immediate aftermath of the separation, Tara adamantly maintained that she was a "good mom." As she reflected on the circumstances of the state intervention, she did not skirt responsibility, "It was really bad judgment." But, she hastened to add, *"I'm not a bad mom."*

Two months later, Tara was granted conditional custody by agreeing to enter a residential substance abuse treatment facility. She was "willing to do anything" to get her kids back, including moving into a place that was "like a prison." When we spoke on the phone a week after the family moved into the facility, Tara was having a difficult time: her three-year-old son was "plowing" through safety gates and running into the hallways, her newborn daughter was "up, like, ten times a night," and the family had been placed in a "freezing corner room" leaving both children sick. Feeling overwhelmed, Tara asked for help. According to her account, she was rebuffed by staff: "There is nothing that we can do [about your room]." The staff also advised her to put her toddler son in day care a few days a week, to which Tara responded, "No, I don't want him to go to day care for at least two weeks, or a week, or something. . . . He doesn't know where he is. He is lost. The kids are friggin' lost."

Over the next few days, her son continued to "act up real bad" and told his mother, "I don't want to be here." Tara again reached out to the staff: "Would someone sit with me and the kids, you know, for a little while and help me out?" Tara recounted that instead of providing support, "They decided to call the state." Tara refused to sign the paperwork for this process: "I was like, 'Fuck you, guys,' and I left [the treatment facility]. And now, [they say that] I am abandoning the kids because I left and I didn't sign the papers." Tara reflected on her situation:

> I am literally fucked. I have nothing. Everything that I have worked for—they are saying that I have abandoned the kids. Why would I go through all of this to walk away? I wouldn't. And it makes me sick to my stomach that there are people that think that I have abandoned my children. Yeah. "You left." Of course, I did. You told me that you are taking my kids for the second time, I am gone. I ain't going to sit around and sign the fucking paper. I mean, honestly, if you lost your kid— and you lost him for the second time because you asked for help. Just because I wanted somebody to talk to [voice trails off]. Of course, they didn't say it, but, of course, they are thinking that I am not mentally stable. I am perfectly fine. I just needed a hand. That is what they are there for. [My husband was] like, "Just talk to them. Just talk to them." I talked to them. And they called DCF [Department of Children and Families].

After leaving the treatment facility, Tara lived out of her car, having been evicted following her arrest:

> I've lost my apartment. I've lost everything. I'm definitely homeless again. . . . I have no clothes. I have nothing. Nothing. I just want to start over. I don't care anymore. I don't care about possessions. I don't fuckin' care. I have worn the same clothes for like, two days. I just—I give up. What more can I do? I am not using drugs. That was their biggest thing. Why did you guys take my kids? Why can't you guys help me? . . . I mean, [the treatment facility] was not safe. It is not a fuckin' safe atmosphere. And I talked to [my caseworker] for a good forty-five minutes. And, she is like, "I understand. These are all really, really, really good points. And we will try to fix it, and this and that." Well, that is their way of fixing it: taking the fuckin' kids.

When I visited Tara in the spring of 2012—nearing the one-year anniversary of the separation from her children—she had made great strides toward "starting over." With the assistance of a private, faith-based philanthropic organization, she was living in a new apartment and had use of a car. Smiling, she told me, "I've been doing really good. I'm going to AA and NA, church every Sunday, church dinners every Friday." She said that her husband "is out of my life now," adding that, "He always enabled me. When I got out of rehab, he was there with methadone in his pocket." She described how, when she had first moved into this new apartment, he "beat the shit out of me for five hours." She obtained a restraining order against him, anticipating that "he'll be going to jail for like eight to sixteen years, 'cause this is his third offense."

Tara gave me a tour of her new apartment, which occupied the second story of a nineteenth-century house. As we made our way through the spacious rooms, I remarked that she had made it "so homey." She smiled knowingly, "I always do." Whether living in a shelter, a motel room, or her own apartment, Tara had a talent for making these spaces *home*. Particularly poignant were the care and attention given to her children's rooms. With the beds made up in colorful linens and toys and books at the ready, one would never guess that these rooms remained empty but for brief visits. Tara was, as ever, expecting the imminent return of her children, explaining: "The issue was [my husband]. Now that he's out of my life, I can have my kids back." For the first year after being separated from her children, it seemed that she was forever on the cusp of getting her kids back.

Two months later, the children remained in state custody, and Tara was like a different person when I picked her up outside of her apartment. Her eyes were heavily rimmed in black eyeliner and mascara, accentuating the flatness of her expression. She asked me to take her to pick up a prescription. As we drove along the winding Vermont road past farmhouses and trailers to the pharmacy, Tara stared straight ahead. The sense of hope and possibility that had infused our visit just two months earlier had vanished. A few weeks later, Tara had "quit the [philanthropic] program" and was living in a homeless shelter. She looked thin and tired when I picked her up outside the shelter. She told me that she was struggling to stay "clean" in this environment. She was hoping to find a job to have "something to do during the day," but her caseworker advised her to "Just concentrate on herself and getting the kids back now." I asked her what she does during the day, and she shook her head, "Just try to keep to myself." Having been alienated from the basic tasks of caring for her young children, Tara struggled with boredom and a lack of routine. With boredom, the gravitational pull of drugs grew stronger. So it did not surprise me when I heard a rumor around the shelter a few weeks later that "Tara was *out of her mind*" on drugs.

When we saw each other next, Tara had just completed a 28-day rehab program and had moved into a motel room. She looked rested. We folded laundry together as she set up house yet again. She told me that she "found God" in rehab, and even though she had no money (and, in fact, did not know how she would pay the bill for her room that night), she was confident that "He'll provide." She proceeded to vent about "*those people*" at the shelter and her need to get away from all the "losers" and "takers" in her life. We spent the afternoon running errands—first a stop at a food pantry followed by a meeting with her parole officer. She was visibly buoyed when her parole officer did not make her "do a urine [test]." Proudly, Tara said, "This is the first time that's ever happened!" We headed back to the motel and chatted as we put groceries away in the kitchenette. When she said that her husband was coming to see her later that night, my heart sank. I asked her how she felt about it, and her reply was nonchalant, "Oh, it'll be fine." Later that evening, my thoughts turned to Tara, and I sent her a text message: "Hey hun. Thinking of u. Take care of yourself." I did not hear from her again for nearly another month.

Tara had moved again when I saw her next, this time into an apartment she was sharing with a roommate. Uncharacteristically, she did not invite me in. She asked if I could take her to the pawn shop: "I wanna sell my ring. I'm *broke*." As we waited at a stoplight, she surprised me when she said that she had not been visiting the kids regularly. As her fingers worried the silver ring, she elaborated that the foster parents—two middle-class professionals—wanted to adopt the children. With exhaustion and resignation in her voice, she said simply, "I don't want to confuse them anymore. I just want them to have a normal life."

I lost contact with Tara when she was incarcerated for drug possession. Tara's parental rights were ultimately terminated, and the children were adopted.

*   *   *

Jim and Hannah were a married couple with a large, blended family[5] who were raising their four children. They were in their forties and White. Jim and Hannah had completed some college and had long work histories in the restaurant industry prior to disabling injuries. Both struggled with chronic physical conditions and reported mental health conditions including depression, anxiety, and PTSD.

"It was just an accident." This simple sentence encapsulates the event that would compel Hannah, her husband Jim, and their children to uproot from a southern state to Vermont in 2007. Jim's accident resulted in a disability that left him unable to work at that time: "I went from the guy working seventy hours a week to basically . . . bedridden." His condition stymied the medical community and, with deep cuts to Medicaid in this southern state, the family moved north to access medical care:

> I couldn't get the testing done there: nobody would pay for it. And I knew we could here. I also knew I'd met two of the neurologists up here that really had an idea of what was going on. They guided my doctor down in [southern state] as to what to do. And I said, "Well, we're wasting our time. Let's go to the source." And, I mean, we were gonna end up homeless there—homeless with no medical insurance. I said, "We need to go."

The family moved with the financial support of their church to access medical care for Jim and their children, several of whom were also contending with chronic health conditions:

> And the church—someone within the church heard about what was going on with us. Someone with a lot of money. And they put up the money to get us up here and pay for a year of rent. And that's why we moved up here more than anything else. . . . And, I mean, all we did was start throwing darts around [medical center] looking for places to live.

They described being advised to move to Vermont (rather than New Hampshire) to access more generous benefits:

> And we finally got the woman from New Hampshire on the phone—one of the counselors. Hannah talked to her about what we were trying to do and what benefits were available. And the woman said, "What are you looking at [in terms of location]?" And Hannah said, "Well, we're looking at Vermont, New Hampshire. . . ." And Hannah didn't even finish the sentence and the counselor said, "Move to Vermont." [laughs] She said just, "Move to Vermont." She goes, "With what you're going through, you'll have better resources, you'll have better support than you would in New Hampshire."

As Hannah and Jim recounted their early months in Vermont, they described having forged new friendships, and this period was narrated as a time of possibility. Hannah said, "There was a point I remember, there was a point for about six months where I seriously thought and entertained the idea and felt like I maybe really could have the ability to go back to school. You know? And I was really excited."

This sense of possibility faded as the family's finances "became a complete disaster." By this time, they had exhausted the philanthropic resources that had enabled their move, and Jim had been advised not to seek employment while he applied for Social Security disability benefits. Their newfound friendships also quickly eroded as Hannah described how her friends had "evaporated." Her voice was tinged with bitterness as she recounted the story: "As soon as the shit hit the fan," when the family was evicted, her friends were unwilling to take them in. "I asked her, 'Can we stay in a tent in the backyard?' This is a person who was my best friend, talked to five times a day, and it's, 'Sorry, can't help you.' . . . They wouldn't let their kids play with my kids. One girl's husband wouldn't let her talk to me anymore. They stopped answering their phones." With nowhere to go and no money to move south, the family moved into Safe Harbor. Jim described this as an intentional choice: "We chose to stay at the [shelter] because the support we needed was finally happening. All of the pieces were coming together in one place."

When shelter staff became concerned that the family was overwhelmed caring for the children, an advocate contacted the child welfare office to inquire about available services. Jim explained: "And they tell her to write a letter [to the Department of Children Youth and Families] describing some of the difficulty so that they can sit down and really get some support going for us. And they turn around and use it against us." Shortly thereafter, their four children—ranging in age from three to eight years—were taken into state custody in Vermont. The separation involved the police and child welfare officials arriving to remove the children from the shelter. The evening is still remembered as "traumatic" among shelter staff. Several months later, Hannah reflected: "What else can we lose? We've already lost everything as far as I'm concerned. . . . My biggest fear is how much am I gonna lose of myself that's never gonna come back?"

Jim and Hannah no longer qualified to stay at the family shelter after their children were taken into custody in the fall of 2009. They moved from the shelter into a pay-by-the-week motel, where they stayed for three months. Despite having a Section 8 subsidized housing voucher, they—like many others—found it difficult to find a landlord willing to "take a chance" on them. They attributed this to the stigma of having been homeless: "We were trying to find housing. And we got denied, and denied, and denied. . . .

They were afraid to put someone in there that was homeless because there
is this fear like, 'Oh, you are homeless. There must be something wrong.'"
The stakes were especially high in their case given that stable housing was
a condition of reunification with their children.

From the motel, they eventually moved into a rental house. As the couple
settled into the house, they described the aftershocks of the family upheaval
manifesting in disorientation to time and the obliteration of routines of
caregiving:

> Well, being a parent now under this circumstance has gotta be the most frustrat-
> ing thing in the world. We walk around—there's so much we need to do. But you
> don't have your own little cues, you know? And I mean, maybe that sounds silly
> but when the kids are there, you have a better schedule. (Jim)

Without the children present to anchor their daily experiences, their actions
took on a phantom-like quality. Efforts to organize possessions and set up
house were oriented toward children who were not there, revealing a razor's
edge between the insistent hope of reunification and the amplification of
their absence:

Jim: With just the two of us here, we find ourselves walking around . . . and
when we do have free time, doing stuff that really doesn't have to be done.
Hannah started organizing toys. And we're both, like, "Why are we doing
this?"

Hannah: Everything's just totally insane—

Jim: Finding the drive, finding the drive. The kids, the kids were my drive. . . .
And with them gone, you just feel alone. . . . There's a huge piece of you
that doesn't know what to do—like, "What am going to do with this right
now?" . . . I know I had the fear if I go around and I start setting everything
else up and making it nice and neat and organized that the other shoe's
gonna drop and something's gonna go wrong. But we're hoping this week-
end that we think we both decided we're gonna really start. Just going ahead
and making the assumption and setting up like we're gonna get ready and
have the kids back here.

The lower level of the house brimmed with black trash bags full of their
family's belongings, having been shuttled across their various moves. Yet
week after week, the bags sat unpacked.

During this time, their days were subsumed by appointments with lawyers, vocational rehabilitation specialists, case managers, and a bevy of

medical and mental healthcare providers (see chapter 4) as they made efforts to meet court mandates for reunification. Despite these efforts, the family remained separated. Yet the couple was hopeful: "[Our primary care physician] goes, 'These are two good people that I think once they get through this, they're gonna come out on the other side of it.' . . . A good part of me knows that it's gonna be okay somehow or another and we'll get through it" (Jim).

But this sense of hope faded a few months later when the reunification was further undermined when they again lost housing. In this case, their landlord refused to make repairs to the rental property to comply with Section 8 regulations, upending the fragile security they had achieved, along with the promise of their children returning. Without housing, it was impossible to bring their children home. The couple felt that the "cards were stacked against them" and described being treated by the court "like criminals": "We've got people questioning every move I make, everything I do" (Jim).

Unable to find housing, they spent the next five months squatting on a wooded hillside, surviving on food stamps and $98 in monthly cash assistance. They continued to engage with countless health, social, and legal services in an ongoing effort to be reunited with their children. Initially, they slept in a tent, where they had regular encounters with mice and a black bear in their camp. During this time, they bathed in a brook, which also served as a makeshift refrigerator. Lacking a car, they walked miles every day to attend appointments with social service providers and to run errands. As the weather turned colder, they moved into an abandoned bus on the property, and Jim fashioned a wood-fired heater. Reflecting on this time, Jim said tenderly to Hannah, "I wasn't going to let you freeze. You know that." Yet the strain of sleeping outside, contending with harsh weather and wildlife, and walking miles every day to attend appointments took its toll on their marriage (see chapter 3).

With the approach of the New England winter, they were grateful to find a rental house and a landlord willing to accept their Section 8 voucher. After moving into the house, Jim and Hannah proudly gave me a tour. Our conversation turned to canopy beds as they described how they planned to set up the children's bedrooms. As they anticipated the nearing court date for the termination of their parental rights, they were confident that the outcome would be in their favor given that they had secured housing: "They [moved to terminate parental rights] before we had the house. . . .

And so my lawyer said that she wouldn't be surprised if they would back off of it." With their housing subsidy capping rent at 30% of income and Jim's return to work, the couple was finally on more stable financial footing. Following the proceeding to terminate their parental rights, they were again confident that the judge's ruling would result in reunification as they described how their lawyers "took charge" and "got in the zone."

Jim and Hannah waited for five months for the judge's ruling and were devastated by the news that their parental rights had been terminated. Hannah's mental health was a key element of the official case reports presented during the hearing. According to Jim, these reports described Hannah as a "sociopath." She was devastated by the descriptions of her "withdrawal" from her children during visitations: "I've been so depressed. It basically said that I'm just a horrible mother." Jim was quick to counter that Hannah's therapist had said that such a response was a "normal defense" given the circumstances. Earlier in their experience, they had described the toll wrought by homelessness as leading to withdrawal and the extinguishment of motivation (see chapter 2). In addition, the case report raised the issue of their financial situation: "It said that Jim and I can't take care of our basic needs." Jim stood up for his legal rights: "You cannot legally discriminate on financial grounds in custody cases. The law is very clear." Yet in the official record, Hannah's withdrawn behavior and their limited resources were used as evidence to cast doubt on their ability to parent.

Jim and Hannah held onto their Section 8 rental house for nearly two years following the termination of their parental rights. When a social service provider pointed out this success and asked them how they had accomplished this, Hannah was adamant: "My home is my top priority. . . . Utilities come last, heat comes last. . . . I do not allow myself—I do not let anything else happen unless my home is taken care of." Jim echoed this: "Being without propane, without hot water, that's just an inconvenience. Keepin' that roof up there is the priority." During this time, Jim landed a job at a local restaurant, which further stabilized their financial situation. Despite the pain of losing the children, it seemed that their situation was improving, a view they shared: "So far, we've been able to succeed, to move on."

When they were subsequently evicted from this property for hoarding, they lost their Section 8 voucher and moved to a market-rate rental in a more remote town. The house was situated off a rutted dirt road and was little more than a cabin, yet it commanded $1,100 for the monthly rent,

reflecting the high cost of living in this rural community. They had no cel-
lular service in this location, and even their landline was susceptible to out-
ages. Despite these challenges, Jim and Hannah enjoyed being surrounded
by nature and established a vast vegetable garden. They were beginning to
feel more financially comfortable with the prospect of combining the income
from Jim's job with Hannah's new disability benefits for a chronic condition.

A point of inflection came when Jim lost his job, sparking a cycle of falling behind on rent. When their old car broke down, they were stranded.
Quotidian tasks of getting groceries, doing laundry, and going to doctor's
appointments became outsized hurdles in daily life. The longer Jim and
Hannah stayed in the remote cabin, the more isolated they became. This
isolation was both physical and existential as they became increasingly
alienated from the routines and norms of community life. Hannah's appearance became unkempt. The woman who, years before, had preened in the
mirror and fussed with frosted pink lipstick now wore the same dirty jeans,
baggy sweatshirt, and trucker cap each time we met. We took to meeting
outside as the house became impassable with piles of their possessions. The
isolation seemed to further fuel depression and heavy alcohol use as beer
cans piled up in the field next to the house. I sat with Jim one late summer
afternoon as he described their situation:

> We're looking at possibly losing the house at the end of the month because our
> lease is up and we owe the landlord money. . . . It feels like after four years of
> finally getting somewhere and feeling more comfortable, and then moving here
> and feeling even more comfortable—boom. Here it goes again. . . . The last few
> weeks have just been fighting depression. I'm terrified of heading back into a
> place I've already been. As much as we've been through, I'm like, "I don't think I
> can do it this time around."

When I asked him if they had considered moving back to the South to
access cheaper housing, he explained that they did not want to move so far
from the children (despite the fact that legally they could have no contact).

Hannah was gripped by a constellation of fear and inertia at the prospect
of losing yet another home. As I sat with her on a late summer afternoon,
she wept. "What are we going to do? I'm lost. Stuck. Numb. Like watching
myself in a movie. You know it's reality, but it's like you're watching yourself."
Hannah's despair was embodied in her increasingly disheveled appearance.
In my fieldnotes from this time, I wrote: *She seemed really out of it today. As*
Hannah was talking, there would be long pauses during which her mouth gaped

open and she seemed very far away. I wondered at the impact of alcohol and the medications she was prescribed for pain management.

As detailed in the opening scene of the book, Jim and Hannah lost their housing when the landlord refused to renew their lease. They were months behind on rent, they had spiraled deeply into alcohol use, and their hoarding behaviors had escalated. Lacking other options, they moved to a motel in a distant town where they rented a tiny efficiency room for $220 per week. Hannah spent long days alone as Jim commuted an hour each way to work shifts at a convenience store. She grew ever more isolated: "I don't want to be in the country. I'm suffocating. . . . Do you know what I would give for human connection?"

Jim returned home from a long shift and found Hannah dead. I still do not know the exact cause. As of this writing, Jim and I have fallen out of touch despite my continued efforts to reach out. Our last communication before he fell silent was on January 15, 2015, when I received a text message at 3 a.m. In the black and white photo, a 20-something Hannah looks directly into the camera, her eyes piercing, her brow furrowed, her mouth slightly open. I'm struck by her gorgeous curly hair, her porcelain skin. Only the eyes are recognizable. Jim captioned the photo: "My baby when I married her. Vermont destroyed her. I'm leaving. Please call."

Madness at the Interface of Loss and Systems of Power

Families in the study interfaced with countless institutions and organizations as they made efforts to meet their survival needs. Engaging with support services is usefully considered as a form of moral engagement through which parents strive to fulfill basic responsibilities of "good" parenthood by accessing needed resources, thus repairing (at least partially) the "failure" of homelessness. Yet by seeking services, parents also sacrifice autonomy and privacy (Tischler et al., 2007). Parents are placed in a double bind as they "parent in public" (Friedman, 2000), and, consequently, "Their parenting is more visible to government and public agencies than that of their middle class counterparts" (Appell, 1998, p. 356; Kay, 2009). In the glare of the professional gaze, parental actions and inactions are titrated out from the flow of daily experience and are recast as evidence of parental fitness. Homeless mothers, like Tara and Hannah, are particularly vulnerable to being stigmatized as inadequate parents (Barrow & Laborde, 2008). This stigma is compounded among parents who experience psychiatric disabilities (National Council on Disability, 2012).

After the initial shock dissipated, the early weeks and months of separation were a time of resolve and optimism for families. There was a sense that a horrible error has been made but that the egregious wrong would soon be righted. At this point, parents had no reason to doubt that the state bureaucracy operated rationally and that regaining custody of their children was assured so long as they complied with the conditions set forth by child welfare officials in their official case plan. Parents made good-faith efforts to comply with these conditions—participating in counseling, consenting to urine screens and staying "clean," securing housing, severing ties with violent partners. In setting up bedrooms for children who were not present, parents sought to reground themselves to domestic rhythms as they awaited the imminent return of their children. As parents navigated systems of power to regain parental rights, they occupied spaces of moral experimentation and striving (Mattingly, 2014), propelled by the hope of reunification with their children. These efforts underscore the "struggle" (Jenkins, 2015b) of lives marked by precarity.

Yet over time, their efforts to "do everything they're asking" were not rewarded; their children never came home. In the eyes of the child welfare system, there was always a need for "further evaluation" or "more clean time," thus prolonging the separations. This is due in large part to the fact that case plans lay out specific activities for parents to do but do not define the goal or outcome measure such that, "Workers don't know what they're asking of families, so families can never achieve it" (S. Kobylenski, personal communication, August 18, 2017). In such experiences, we hear echoes of the "institutionally and politically engendered double binds" identified by Janis Jenkins (1991, p. 157) in her discussion of the state construction of affect among Salvadoran refugees.

Similar to the political asylum seekers described by Bridget Haas (2017), parents separated from their children spent their days and weeks *waiting*. Haas argues that a life subsumed by waiting provokes a subjective and temporal state of "existential limbo" that perpetuates suffering and generates new forms of trauma (2017, p. 88). In my time with Tara, Hannah, and Jim, I observed how the loss of children produced tectonic shifts in parents' ways of being in the world as life lost coherence and structure. Under these conditions, the existential moorings of family life were shattered as everyday life was reoriented away from caregiving. As the state prolonged separations, parents were stripped of a principal grounding and motivating force in their lives.

This state of existential limbo for the families in the study had dire consequences for their capacities as parents. The traumatic rupture of intersubjective familial ties resulted in the gradual erosion and eventual loss of parental selves. As the weeks of separation stretched into months and the months into years, Hannah's "biggest fear" was realized: "How much am I gonna lose of myself that's never gonna come back?" Tara came to embody the stereotype of the "homeless addict." The experiences of the families in this chapter thus call attention to unintended consequences of intervention.

Such devastation would likely be interpreted within the child welfare system as confirmation of the status of these individuals as "unfit" parents. I argue instead that these subjective effects point to a form of madness induced by navigating state systems of power in the wake of traumatic loss. I am not asserting that mental health or substance use disorders were caused by engagement with the child welfare system. For both of the families described in this chapter, mental health vulnerabilities and addiction were present prior to the removal of their children. Instead, I seek to call attention to how institutional systems, including state child welfare agencies, potentially worsen the course and outcome of mental illness and substance abuse and, through demoralization, erode parental capacities. The loss of parental selves and transformation into "bad" parents occurred within the context of a state system that amplified these families' vulnerabilities. The system not only failed to address cycles of trauma (Liu et al., 2021) and conditions of structural violence (Farmer, 1996) among families experiencing homelessness, mental health, and substance use challenges but may, in fact, be "traumatic reenactments masquerading as benign practice" (Harris & Fallot, 2001, p. 9). The time apart from children did not "fix" these parents (Appell, 1998).[6] When parental rights were ultimately terminated, hope reveals itself as a form of delusion. Hope "in the face of structural violence and foreclosed opportunity . . . may not always be a positive thing" (Jenkins & Csordas, 2020, p. 221) just as "imagining a certain future [can] be emotionally and psychically dangerous" (Haas, 2017, p. 91). After losing responsibility for the care of their children[7] and experiencing the contradictions and broken promises of a punitive child welfare system,[8] these parents see life itself unravel.

Systemic constraints within the child welfare system manifest in limited funding and caseloads far exceeding recommended standards (Crist & Bech, 2018). Lacking time and funding, child welfare offices in Vermont have few resources beyond the removal of children and thus err on the side of "not taking chances" (S. Kobylenski, personal communication, August 18, 2017; see also Walsh, 2016). As Michael Lipsky (1980/2010) has argued in relation to "street-level bureaucrats" such as child welfare caseworkers, "high caseloads, episodic encounters, and the constant press of decisions force them to act without even being able to consider whether an investment in searching for more information would be profitable" (p. 29). Constraints within the child welfare system place overworked and underpaid caseworkers in paradoxical roles, as this legal aid lawyer observed:

> Listening to them talk about people, it does seem odd—like they're both in a prosecutorial and supportive role. And it seems like these nice-enough people get put into this role of being super judgmental. Like, "Oh, this person is doing well, and we're supporting her. This person isn't doing well, and we're taking her kids." I just think it's hard to play both sides effectively.

Building from the lawyer's observation, case workers are operating within institutional structures that blur the line between the work of family support and the work of family surveillance and separation. Moreover, child welfare investigations "interpret conditions of poverty—lack of food, insecure housing, inadequate medical care—as evidence of parental unfitness" (Roberts, 2022, p. 21). The risk-averse stance of the Vermont child welfare system arguably misapprehends harm in the case of neglect and so-called risk of harm cases given compelling evidence that children "on the margin of care" fare better over time if they remain with parents rather than enter the foster system (Doyle, 2007, p. 1584). This compels attention to the "foundational logic" of the child welfare system that emphasizes removal of children over support of families amid a "façade of benevolence" (Roberts, 2022, p. 23).

Reimagining Alternate Endings

I came to know Tara, Jim, and Hannah as deeply human—flawed, loving, and striving for their families. Winding back the clock as I poured over years of field notes and transcripts of conversations, I was jolted by the lucidity and functionality of these parents at earlier points in time. My own memories of them as worn down and difficult to follow and my suspicions of alcohol or drug use represented an endpoint of a process years in the making. The traumatic losses endured by these families set in motion a trajectory that left them ultimately embodying the "unfit" parents that they were accused of being, compelling consideration of the impact of custody losses on the course and outcome of mental health experiences. Their downward trajectories were not predetermined.

Close attention to the experiences of families unfolding over time reveals critical junctures where it might have been possible to alter the course of these families' experiences. In considering alternate endings, the specific form of ethnographic engagement that I term an *anthropology of the intimate* provides unique opportunities to bear witness to strengths that might otherwise be invisible to formal institutions. It also raises questions regarding the conditions of possibility for recovery for families marginalized by the systems of care in place for mental illness, substance abuse, homelessness, and poverty. What if Hannah's friends had offered shelter instead of "evaporating"? What if evictions had been avoided? What if intensive mental health and substance use services had nourished and upheld these families instead of being mobilized punitively? What if parents' moral striving had been recognized and supported by health, legal, and social service professionals instead of eroded?

These questions counter the primacy of individualism in mental health recovery (cf. Myers, 2015) and compel recognition of the role of systems and communities in cultivating conditions more (or less) conducive to recovery. Periods of stability and strength were not acknowledged and seized upon by the range of service professionals in these families' lives. For example, when Tara was engaged in peer recovery efforts, had secured stable housing, and had a supportive community assisting her, child welfare professionals did not build on her efforts. Similarly, when Jim and Hannah had found affordable housing and were more financially stable following Jim's return to work, these significant changes in their circumstances did not lead to reunification with their children. Even when, as is possible in these cases, termination of parental rights may be warranted, the experiences of these two families raise the question: are there ways to engage compassionately with parents to recognize profound loss and lessen the trauma of dismantling families?

6 Toward Security Following Homelessness

In this chapter, I build on earlier discussions of families' ongoing efforts as they "strive for ordinary" amid conditions of precarity. Such striving manifests in a range of ways—deciding to change jobs in the hope of finding a more regular schedule; creating family traditions that foster continuity despite mobility or turmoil; cultivating connections to place and home by tending vegetable gardens, keeping a tidy house, or displaying family photographs. These efforts offer a strong counternarrative to prevailing discourses of deficit for rural families living in poverty. Yet, as earlier chapters demonstrate, individual efforts alone are not sufficient to offer sustained protection from the myriad social and structural forces of disruption in families' lives—eviction, relapse, unemployment, isolation, and poverty.

By engaging with families over a long temporal horizon, I have witnessed the unfolding of their experiences against an "unknown future" (Mattingly, 1994, p. 820). From the vantage of looking back over more than a decade, it becomes possible to see the catalysts of both strife and stability in their lives. Whereas previous chapters have detailed the fundamental insecurity, missed opportunities, and unintended consequences of care endured by families, this chapter examines how some families have been able to move toward greater security over time. I argue that the confluence of structural supports and the capacities of families create possibilities for greater security and opportunities for families to engage meaningfully with existing services and resources. When I use the terms *stability* and *security*, I am referring to both material resources (access to housing and basic needs) as well as the lived, felt sense of security articulated by families and encapsulated in an affective vocabulary of "calm," "stable," "peaceful," or, more simply, "we're okay" (cf. Shaw, 2004). By bridging both the material and the subjective experiences of security, the orientation taken in this chapter aims to avoid pathologizing mobility or houselessness. Mobility is not necessarily productive of distress. Rather, distress manifests at the intersection of material conditions of poverty and their consequences for lived experiences of social rejection, shame, and diminishment of hope.

Over the course of this research, all families experienced periods of stability. For some, like Abigail, this was measured in months as she moved between settings of greater and lesser support. Others, including Nancy, Tara, and Jim and Hannah, experienced longer periods of stability that were eventually upended by divorce, eviction, exacerbations of substance use and mental illness, and involvement in the child welfare and criminal justice systems. Barbara's family stands out as an exception to these patterns. Following their nine-month stay at Safe Harbor, Barbara, her long-term partner, and her children have had stable housing for more than a decade. Despite a history of serious substance use and trauma, Barbara has not experienced major mental health or addiction challenges during this time. This does not mean that life has been easy for Barbara—far from it. Rather, she and her family have been able to weather the challenges that they have faced and have not had their lives severely disrupted. Following my consideration of Barbara's experience, I turn to the significant change in Nancy's experience that occurred midway through the research. Similar to others in the study, Nancy had endured ongoing housing insecurity in the first five years that I knew her family. But in 2015, following another period of homelessness, her family gained access to subsidized housing through a supportive housing program in Vermont. She and her two children have remained in this apartment for over five years.

Family Portrait: Enduring Security Following Homelessness

When I met Barbara, she was in her early 40s and was raising two teenaged daughters and a 10-year-old son. Barbara was in a long-term relationship with her partner, Evan. The family had moved into Safe Harbor in the summer of 2009 after becoming homeless in Florida. They had moved out of state to pursue job opportunities and a lower cost of living. But, as Barbara reflected, "Things didn't work out that way. When we left [New England], I thought that the jobs were going to be there, but they weren't." Moreover, she was grieving the loss of her father, whom she had adored. Speaking about that complicated time, she noted:

We just weren't in the right mindset. We had just been through too much. And we were not equipped to deal with anything—with any kind of responsibility. We had just frivolously spent money like there was no tomorrow. It was just very foolish. Neither one of us had any kind of skill. We just made a lot of mistakes down there.

In the first few months of getting to know Barbara, the narrative of her family's pathway into homelessness remained vague. It seemed to reflect a confluence of circumstances involving grief and a swift move away from New England as the family sought opportunities that, ultimately, were nonexistent in the earliest months of the Great Recession. Many years later, I learned that the family's housing crisis had also been precipitated by substance use (see chapter 2). When the family returned to New England, they found they had nowhere to go:

> We came here [to Vermont] and were looking for housing and couldn't find it right away—or jobs. I was in a motel. I had looked in the phone book under "service" or something like that. I called a place in Brattleboro, and they had referred me there [to Safe Harbor.] And I called them because I was out of money, out of—I didn't know where we were going to sleep at night.

Barbara quickly forged a trusting relationship with one of the shelter staff members:

> I mean, I really got close to [shelter staff member]. She's just—there was something so—I don't know. She just had a way about her. Just connected really quick with her when I first got there. I remembered just calling on the phone and being so *desperate* to get into someplace instead of, you know, staying in the car. And there was her voice on the other end of the phone and sitting at the intake. And you don't forget things, or *I* don't, of people who have helped you in ways that basically my own family wouldn't even have helped. So it's really kind of special to me.

With the support of Safe Harbor, Barbara soon found a job and received a subsidized housing voucher. Yet, like others in the study, despite holding a housing voucher, it took many months to find an apartment and a landlord willing to rent to her family. She described the process during one of our drives together:

> Well, I got my housing voucher last week. It was last Wednesday or Thursday, actually. And I am working with a lady that has a house in [New Hampshire town]. Well, it's an apartment. They got together with [the director of Safe Harbor] because you have to be, like, sponsored. And so, [the director] sponsored us. That's because we would be neat and clean, and they knew that we would be a good fit in there. I have been doing my paperwork on it since probably October. So, you know, it is just such a waiting game, right now. And it's just—it's just I want it so bad. . . .

And so, we're waiting to hear from her. That's because she had to go up to the board of directors to see if they would take Section 8. So that happened on Wednesday night, and I still haven't heard anything back. . . . So it just seems like you are always waiting on something else either paperwork or [trails off]. I think that is the most frustrating part of looking for housing in this area. You really have to jump through hurdles to get into a place. That is, even if you have the greatest credit. They are doing so many checks upon checks to see—it is really to weigh their decision out. And it's really a tiring, painstaking process, you know? It's really frustrating.

In this rural setting with limited housing supply and high demand, landlords were selective and cautious about prospective tenants. As many families experienced, landlords appeared especially risk-averse toward renting to those with a history of homelessness. Barbara benefitted from the shelter director's willingness to sponsor the family as a "good fit." Being a "good fit" included Barbara's knack for tidiness, her persistence and organization during the housing search, her steady, supportive relationship with Evan, and the fact that they were both employed. In this way, Barbara and her family embodied "deservingness" (cf. Snell-Rood & Carpenter-Song, 2018; Willen, 2012) and, as such, were positioned to counter the stigma associated with a history of homelessness.

After their long wait, the family moved into a subsidized apartment near a town center in New Hampshire. The apartment occupied part of the second story of a home that had been converted to a multifamily dwelling. Shortly after they had moved in, Barbara described the significance of their new home:

I still can't say enough about how nice it is to be out of the shelter. . . . And, you know, just to sit back and not keep hearing the other people. I get up in the morning and just look at my kids and Evan. I just—I can't even explain it, really. Because it's still kind of—you know, sometimes when I'm at work I think, "I'm going to go home." You know, going home. And I keep saying it to myself because it's just surreal. You know? After being there [at the shelter] for *nine* months. And I keep saying, "*Nine* months." You know it's such—it's such a long time. . . . I mean, the apartment is not—it's not the greatest thing inside, but to me it's just like a little heaven, you know, really. I guess unless you've been in the situation when you live there [at the shelter], it's so hard to make somebody understand what it's truly like. I mean, when [the landlord] called me and told me, "You *can* move in on this day," I was like, "Oh, my God!" Just tears coming out my eyes. I was just like, "Oh finally, finally!"

For Barbara, leaving the shelter was a key milestone in her efforts toward self-sufficiency. Throughout the time I have known her, she has ascribed to deeply held values of self-reliance. As discussed in earlier chapters, this orientation often manifested in Barbara's criticisms of others. In contrast to others at Safe Harbor who "leave the shelter and then they're back, like, every day for food, bread, whatever," Barbara "couldn't wait to get out of there and never come back through those doors again."

Over the course of their first year in the apartment, Barbara held several different jobs, and Evan worked steadily. At one point when Barbara lost her job, she worried about their ability to afford rent. She held off paying utility bills to prioritize the rent payment, as she stated, "I don't care about anything else." At the time, they owed $180 in rent. When Evan received a check in payment for odd jobs he had done at Safe Harbor, Barbara took swift action: "I immediately said, 'We gotta get a money order for rent today.'" While Barbara was deeply grateful for housing following their experience of homelessness, she also viewed this apartment as a temporary place for her family:

ECS: You don't see this as a long-term place?

Barbara: No, I don't. I would like to have a place, Elizabeth, that has a little yard. You know, just something like that, but we don't have that. You know—and don't get me wrong. I am grateful to have the place, but when things go wrong [with the apartment], they are just not, not too quick [to fix things].

Nearing the one-year anniversary of moving in, the rent was raised substantially. Barbara thought that the new figure reflected an error in how their income had been calculated for the subsidy:

Barbara: I want them to put us in the proper bracket that we should be in. I don't want them to be judging and putting an income that they think we are making and we are not.

ECS: So, I'm still not totally sure [I understand]. What are they basing that off of?

Barbara: They are basing this rent off right now. They are saying that our income went over $4,000, okay? So they are taking what [Evan] would make for a whole year. It's because he only started working there in June. So they are taking, like—this is, like, here is this person—here is what you would make in a year. So that is now where they put our income at. So it brings it up $4,000 dollars from what was originally [stated]. And there we have it at like eighteen [thousand dollars]. That is okay. Except that they turned around and added like five grand on there for like a penalty or whatever. I don't understand all of it, you know. So we have ourselves at that bracket. And I was kind of disturbed by it. That is because they make it sound as if

you are trying to keep something from them, which couldn't be further
from the truth, you know.

Navigating rigid eligibility rules for benefits and subsidies was a common
challenge for families in the study. As in Barbara's experience, there was
often little warning when benefits would be cut due to changes in income or
bureaucratic errors. Although she did not fully understand the reason behind
the change in rent, which more than doubled their monthly payment, Barbara had little choice but to do her best to cobble together resources to make
partial, good-faith payments of the amount due. This prompted her to inten-
sify her search for different housing:

> I am in my head thinking about the numbers, too. I'm thinking everything is
> going to balance itself. To come up and look at us, we are not living any—you see
> some people who are living on assistance or whatever, they live better than you
> and I. But when I think of this place here, it's not worth that much money now
> that I have to pay that much. It is not worth it. There is no way. When you don't
> have things insulated properly and things like that. Things start to fall apart.

She continued, describing some of her hopes for a different place:

> It has got to be something where heat is included. I would rather have it all
> with my rent and know that we are okay. You know what I mean? Even if I had
> to pay the extra, at least it's in there, and I don't have to have that worry. It's
> because when you have kids and stuff. My bedroom and [my daughter's] is nice
> and warm. And [my son's room] is like an ice box. It is so cold in there. . . . Some
> people own property, and they don't want to put any money in it, Elizabeth.
> They just want to collect the money that is due for rent or whatever.

About a month later, Barbara and her family were settling into a new
apartment subsidized by their newly "portable" Section 8 voucher. Families
considered a portable voucher to be a coveted resource because it allowed
them the flexibility to move without risking losing their subsidy.[1] The
apartment was part of a small complex of well-kept, white clapboard buildings that blended easily into the small New Hampshire town. Barbara gave
me a tour ("I want to show you the place"), and I was struck by the unit's
high ceilings and large windows. The bright winter sun shone through the
blinds, casting a pattern of shadows across the laminate wood floors. This
property, owned and managed by a local housing trust, was in strikingly
better condition than the properties owned by private landlords that other
families in the study lived in. As Barbara described it:

> It's the nicest place that we have had. It is just great. Everything just seems to work
> wonderfully. And, you know, the people that are there, they're friendly. I'm quiet,

anyways. But, you know, they are nice. And it's just a whole different atmosphere compared to the other one. It just kind of overwhelms me when I think about it.

The new apartment, with its fresh paint and sun-filled rooms, seemed to materialize the sense of possibility that Barbara articulated:

> I have a lot of promise for the future. I really do. I've been just with a new zest. I don't know what you want to call it. I just feel different about the New Year. I do. It takes a long time to try to come out from everything that you have gone through so that you don't make some of the mistakes that you have made prior. And that includes money and learning how to handle it and to be able to pay bills. You have to figure out how we are going to make this work now.

During this time, Evan worked steadily at the same local business. Barbara also worked regularly, although she tended to cycle through jobs after a few months (see chapter 3). The jobs they held were often challenging because of physical demands or difficult interpersonal dynamics. Despite these common challenges of low-wage work, their ability to combine income enabled greater financial security compared to families headed by single parents. In addition, Evan's steady work provided a cushion during brief periods when Barbara was between jobs. Beyond the greater financial security afforded by their partnership, Evan's presence in the family was positive and supportive, unlike many of the relationships among younger women in the study, as Barbara described: "He means the world to me. I couldn't ask for anything better than what he knows. He's wonderful to me. To the children. Just a very good heart and a good soul."

Yet despite these advantages, Barbara was well aware that the security her family experienced was fragile. After pursuing additional training for a job in healthcare, she faced the reality of high-interest student debt that wiped out her tax refund annually. We had many conversations over the years about how "crazy" rents are in the region. Knowing that market-rate housing would be out of reach, Barbara was skilled at the balancing act of working while also maintaining access to housing and healthcare subsidies. She worked diligently with staff from the housing trust to ensure that paperwork was updated and filed on time so as not to jeopardize her family's eligibility for the apartment. Unlike the other families with whom I worked, Barbara and Evan never faced the prospect of losing their home.

In addition to the availability of material resources through steady employment coupled with consistent subsidies, this family's stability was also conditioned by Barbara's specific capacities and subjective orientations. Barbara responded to her family's struggles through her strong orientation toward

self-reliance and her deep religious faith. While the New England bootstrap mentality was defeating for many, Barbara vigorously embraced this
cultural orientation. One day, as she reflected on her time at Safe Harbor,
she recounted, "One of the things I said to the lady who runs the place, 'If I
ran this place, one of the greatest satisfactions I would ever get is not seeing
these people again because it would show me that they're self-sufficient.'"
As detailed in chapter 4, Barbara was skeptical of formal institutions, including healthcare and social services, and expected that people should take
care of problems on their own. Personal responsibility and restraint were
primary threads in the fabric of her experience: "If I couldn't pay for it, I
did without it."

Barbara's adherence to the bootstrap mentality appeared to spark a sense
of agency and possibility for a better future. She dreamed of one day moving away from the Northeast. The warm weather and lower cost of living
beckoned from southern states. Over the course of the research, she took
community college courses in the hope of moving beyond jobs that were
"just mundane." She encouraged her children to "get an education" so they
would not be limited to "meager wages." In the midst of the hard work of
raising her family, Barbara actively cultivated a positive orientation. At one
point, she shared a few things that she had recently thumbtacked on her
"happy wall." Amid the smiling faces of babies and colorful flowers cut out
from magazines were several quotes, such as "In the end, the materialist
project is a lie that may fill our homes, but will leave us hopelessly empty"
and "Happiness is headed your way."

Barbara also found comfort in her religious faith, which she practiced
daily through reading scripture and listening to religious radio programs.
Her faith amplified her positive orientation and reinforced a sense of security as she anticipated her family's future: "I know that God will take care of
all of us. You put your faith in him, and it'll all work out. And that's what
I've done and gives me the strength."

I have now known Barbara for over a decade. As she faces the future, she
and Evan are "empty nesters." The children are all working, pursuing additional education and training, or raising families of their own. She has been
working in a local market for over two years. It is within walking distance
from her apartment, which means she no longer has to worry about unreliable cars or driving on snowy roads to get to work. Although their future is
unknown (cf. Mattingly, 1994), as it is for us all, they appear positioned for
continuing stability and security.

Conditions of Security

Barbara's experience illuminates the individual capacities and structural supports that combined to facilitate enduring (though fragile) security. The circumstances under which her family's trajectory began were similar to those of other families in the study—the loss of housing in the wake of family disruption, unemployment, and the economic fallout of addiction. Yet, after exiting Safe Harbor, the trajectories of these families diverged, and, unlike the chronic housing insecurity endured by the other four families in the study, Barbara, Evan, and the children never again faced the threat of losing their housing. Between 2010, when they left Safe Harbor, and the present, they have moved twice and have maintained the same apartment for the past decade.

What was different about this family's experience? Like a few others in the study, Barbara and her family gained immediate access to subsidized housing after exiting Safe Harbor. Consequently, her family avoided the high market rents in the region, and the housing subsidy ensured that their rent would not exceed 30% of their income. This structural support was foundational to her family's ability to meet its basic needs within the financial constraints of low-wage work. Yet this experience was not unique to Barbara; other families also had access to subsidized housing over the course of the research. But, as detailed in previous chapters, three of the families lost their subsidized housing over time. For Abigail, as a young mother raising small children, the isolation of living in an apartment far from family and friends proved untenable, and she subsequently moved out in search of greater social support yet sacrificed her housing subsidy in the process. Tara also grew increasingly lonely and bored over time. Returning to her hometown, she struggled to distance herself from old friends with whom she had used drugs. An acute need for childcare precipitated reconnecting with this network, and she was drawn back into substance use. Ultimately, an encounter with law enforcement resulted in the removal of her children and also the swift loss of her home. Jim and Hannah were evicted from their home of two years because of hoarding, resulting in the loss of their Section 8 voucher.

By contrast, Barbara's family did not experience isolation or the exacerbation of mental illness or substance use. Temperamentally, Barbara enjoyed "keeping to myself" and spent her days working, reading, or taking walks along the trails close to her apartment complex. Her supportive relationship with Evan also guarded against loneliness and boredom. In addition, despite a history of trauma and substance use, Barbara did not experience mental health problems or relapse during the time of the research. These dimensions of her past experiences were not key elements of her identity. She did not consider herself to be a person "in recovery," nor did she participate in mental or behavioral health services during the time I knew her.

Barbara and her family experienced struggles over the years, but they did not experience any major crises following their period of homelessness. Together, she and Evan were able to weather financial strain by combining wages and subsidies to maximize their family's financial security amid difficult and capricious low-wage work. In addition, because her children were adolescents and she had a partner, Barbara did not require childcare. These circumstances facilitated her ability to take jobs with unpredictable schedules that were untenable for single mothers raising young children. Except for brief periods of unemployment after leaving a job, Barbara worked continuously throughout the time of the research. She may have had greater employment opportunities because of her efforts to gain additional training as well as her own habits of meticulous self-care and social graces that enabled her to "pass" as middle class.

What are the lessons to take from Barbara's experiences? Clearly, access to affordable housing was the key structural determinant of her family's security. Barbara and Evan were able to build from this essential material resource to more fully leverage their social and personal strengths over time. Moreover, their security was not disrupted by mental health crises or substance use relapses. Looking at the experiences of other families, it is possible to imagine a far different trajectory for Barbara, Evan, and the children had they faced the pressures of market-rate housing, low-wage work, and the need for childcare or if they had experienced major mental health or addiction challenges in the intervening years. Yet if the main lesson is that families with fewer needs fare better over time, this seems unsatisfactory to the task of envisioning a broader, more enduring security for families marginalized by poverty and experiencing complex needs.

To offer a more nuanced perspective, I turn to consider the movement toward security among Nancy and her children. In the first five years following their exit from Safe Harbor, Nancy and her two children faced chronic housing insecurity, as detailed in chapter 3. When they returned to Vermont in 2015 after living out of state for a year, however, this marked a point of inflection in this family's experience. In the family portrait below, I describe the dimensions of greater stability and security for Nancy and her children.

Family Portrait: Toward Security Following Homelessness

A year after uprooting from the Northeast with high hopes and an overnight drive to Georgia, Nancy and her children had become homeless again. The promise of support from friends had frayed as relationships grew tense. Once again, in a refrain common to this family, they could no longer double up and were left with nowhere to go. After a brief stint in a Georgia shelter, Nancy made the decision to return to New England.

After returning to Vermont, Nancy reengaged with her previous case manager at Safe Harbor, Jamie. With Jamie's help, Nancy qualified for a supportive housing voucher through a partnership between the shelter and the state of Vermont. Shortly thereafter, the family moved to a subsidized apartment that capped rent at 30% of her income. This marked the first time that Nancy was not paying market-rate rent for housing. The apartment was located close to one of the main towns in the Upper Valley and was situated on the route of the region's free bus line. With easy access to transportation and with her children settling into predictable school schedules, Nancy was able—for the first time since I had known her—to look for paid work. She quickly found a job at a dollar store and enjoyed the work environment: "I can be myself. They don't mind me being a smartass." She stayed at that job for nearly a year and was promoted to assistant manager, which proved to be a double-edged sword. While she appreciated the (slightly) higher pay and recognition of her hard work, she also began to feel overwhelmed by the greater responsibility and expectation of working longer hours, including more evenings and weekends. She was initially able to juggle favors with neighbors to watch the kids, but this arrangement was unsustainable, and she ultimately decided to leave the job.

Reflecting on this decision a few weeks later, Nancy commented, "Not having a job—it's killing my anxiety and everything and my depression. I'm not really depressed, but I'm sleeping a lot. So then I don't sleep at night." She continued, describing how she missed the structure of her routine: "I'd put the kids on the bus, and then I'd come back here and get ready for work and go off to work. I need to find a job. I'm going crazy with nothing to do. I'm so desperate I even applied at Walmart." The entropic force of boredom was manifest in days passed in front of the television smoking pot, in the growing chaos of "stuff" in the apartment, and in the incremental worsening of Nancy's depression and anxiety.

Yet even with the setback of unemployment and ensuing boredom and mental health challenges, Nancy was profoundly aware of positive changes in her family's life: "The kids. They're doing excellent this year in school, and things seem a lot better with them. We've been stable for a year now, and we don't plan on moving at all." Nancy's plan not to move has been realized. The family has lived in this apartment for five years—the longest stretch in a single place in the decade that I have known them. Nancy has worked during most of this time. Her children, Emily and David, have been supported by a network of teachers, mental health specialists, coaches, and advocates. They are engaged in their community, participating in school sports and music programs and also attending summer camps.

The family is visited regularly by case managers who stop by to drop off food and to check in with Nancy. Unlike her interactions with various "workers" earlier in the study, Nancy appeared at ease with these service providers, who, in turn, seemed to accept the family's circumstances and to recognize strength amid ongoing challenges. Nancy's transition to a different case manager a few years ago went smoothly. Over time, she has grown incrementally more comfortable with engaging in mental health services. Both children have worked with therapists for several years, and, recently, Nancy has been seeing a therapist via telehealth. She appreciated being able to talk with someone "close to my age" from the comfort of her home: "I'll be on my bed, smoking a cigarette." Her experience of and orientation toward therapy have shifted over time. While she was previously deeply critical of therapists (see chapter 4), Nancy described her comfort with her new therapist, elaborating about how "It's not all about talking about problems. Sometimes, we just catch up, talk about my life. It's cool." Outside of formal services, Nancy is supported by—and supports—a close neighbor. They cook together several times a week, and her neighbor is available to help with the children. Nancy described their connection in this way: "We've been through the same shit."

As detailed in chapter 3, Nancy has not always had such consistent or supportive social connections. Recently, she has been intentional about "cutting certain people out of my life" and described her resentment over "giving people a couch to sleep on, food, being their therapist." She told me that things are much "calmer" now and that she is enjoying shifting her focus to "just me and the kids." After being unemployed for over a year because of the COVID-19 pandemic and the need to care for the children during remote schooling, Nancy looked forward to returning to work when schools reopened. During the pandemic, she was buoyed by infusions of resources from the federal stimulus program and the expansion of welfare benefits.[2] These resources were essential during this period of extended unemployment, and she proudly noted, "I haven't needed to ask my mom for anything."

Nancy and her family have endured ongoing struggles over the past five years—unemployment, mental health challenges, and precarious relationships. Their housing, though stable, is substandard. Several years ago, a portion of the ceiling in David's room collapsed, revealing black mold. Nancy remains hopeful that they will one day find a three-bedroom apartment so that she does not need to sleep in the living room. Despite experiencing threats to their stability that in the past would have precipitated a housing crisis, the family's ongoing access to affordable housing has enabled continued, though fragile, security.

Conditions of Security Revisited

The experiences of these two families underscore that access to affordable housing is the principal condition of security for families that have experienced homelessness and housing insecurity. In Barbara's case, she and her family gained access to this essential resource immediately after exiting Safe Harbor. Their trajectory has been one of continued stability over time. Nancy and her family, by contrast, endured five years of instability and mobility before gaining access to a subsidized apartment. Since then, they have experienced ongoing threats to their stability. Absent the stable foundation of affordable housing, it is likely that unemployment, mental health exacerbations, or shifts in social support would have plunged Nancy's family into another housing crisis.

As noted earlier in the chapter, it is possible that Barbara, Evan, and the children fared especially well over time because they had fewer needs and could more fully leverage a combination of structural supports and individual capacities. Nancy's experience broadens the frame to facilitate insight into conditions of security in the context of deep and persistent challenges because she continued to experience many dimensions of fundamental insecurity and yet remained stable. In relation to other families in the study for whom periods of stability in affordable housing were eventually disrupted, *What was different about Nancy's experience? Why was she able to weather the threats to her family's security?*

Nancy's experience highlights the confluence of structural supports and particular subjective orientations that created possibilities for greater security. For Nancy, affordable housing was the key structural support that conditioned her family's movement toward security. Beyond this crucial material resource, in Nancy's experience we can see that her own subjective orientations to sociality and shift toward openness to engaging with services were crucial to facilitating greater security for her family. Regarding sociality, Nancy had always maintained a network of friends and associates that enabled a fragile survival and just-in-time access to scarce resources. In addition, this network protected Nancy from the impress of isolation experienced by others in the study. Yet this sociality alone was insufficient to catalyze a more robust security in the absence of stable and affordable housing. When coupled with subsidized housing, Nancy's orientation to sociality facilitated connections to resources, friendship, and opportunities for the family to be more integrated in their community, which consequently augmented material security with a subjective sense of connection and belonging, elements critical to recovery and "the ability to be recognized as a 'good' person in a way that makes possible intimate connections to others" (Myers, 2015, p. 13).

Over time, Nancy grew more open to engaging with social services, case management, and mental health treatment. Unlike Barbara, who limited her use of professional services after leaving Safe Harbor, Nancy and her children became deeply engaged in a range of services following their return to Vermont in 2015. This process began when Nancy was able to rekindle her relationship with her previous Safe Harbor case manager, Jamie, with whom she had developed a deep trust over the years. Jamie embodied continuity of care—always "showing up" whenever Nancy needed her support. With Jamie's assistance, Nancy accessed her supportive housing voucher. Supportive housing programs are designed to combine stable housing with intensive wrap-around services. It is important to recall from chapter 5 that *more* services do not always yield better outcomes for families. Rather, Nancy's experience offers insight into characteristics of services that are subjectively experienced as supportive and that, over time, contribute to families' capacities to address longstanding and emergent challenges. In Nancy's experience in supportive housing services, vulnerabilities are responded to with support and compassion, not surveillance and judgment. Her case manager stops by with food and will help Nancy to clean and organize her apartment before housing inspections. This stands in stark contrast to how professionals interacted with Tara, Jim, and Hannah (see chapter 5). The case managers and mental health professionals now involved in this family's life do not demand that Nancy "prove" her fitness or worth as a parent. In this way, the supportive housing services recognize and augment Nancy's strengths in the context of ongoing struggle.

In this chapter, I have focused on how some families have moved toward greater security over time. For both Barbara and Nancy, gaining access to affordable housing was a crucial determinant of their families' growing stability. They were both able to build from a foundation of stable and affordable housing to amplify their individual strengths. Together, these two families point to common conditions needed for security and underscore the diversity in trajectories toward stability. Barbara and Nancy highlight the heterogeneity of families' needs following experiences of homelessness and housing insecurity. Whereas Barbara continued to distance herself from professional services, Nancy and her children became more engaged with a range of social and mental health services over time through a supportive housing model. Grounded in these families' experiences, I argue that it is the confluence of particular subjective orientations and structural supports that create possibilities for greater security and opportunities for families to more meaningfully engage with existing services and resources, including affordable housing, healthcare, work, education, and community supports. This view disrupts the bootstrap mentality in rural New England by underscoring meaningful recovery from the assaults of homelessness and poverty as a deeply social process, linked to institutional, political, and economic systems cultivating conditions that support families' efforts toward "the good life" (Mattingly, 2014; Myers, 2015). These families' trajectories have been one of incremental improvement akin to the subjective experience of recovery described by Janis Jenkins and Elizabeth Carpenter-Song (2005). This reminds us that families' trajectories are nonlinear and entail daily "struggle" (Jenkins, 2015b; Jenkins & Csordas, 2020). Moreover, a longitudinal perspective grounded in more than a decade of intimate ethnography facilitates the capacity to recognize strength in the midst of seriously disrupting and disabling forces. There is a clear need for families to have access to structural supports and compassionate supportive services that can augment their everyday efforts to build a more secure future for their families.

7 Conclusion

Rural New England is well positioned to more robustly meet the needs of families living in poverty. The economic, educational, and service resources that exist in this setting offer promising conditions for becoming a national model for addressing the intersection of housing, mental health, and substance use in rural communities. Yet, to date, this potential has not been fully realized. As detailed in earlier chapters, for many families, daily life was shadowed by fundamental insecurity that manifests in chronic housing insecurity, the difficulty and instability of low-wage work, geographic and social isolation in rural areas, and fragile relationships. Against the backdrop of fundamental insecurity, families navigated through the rural landscape of care to meet their survival needs. Although these encounters were intended to offer support, there were significant missed opportunities to meaningfully engage families, and, consequently, many remained tenuously and haphazardly engaged in care. For some, engagement with professional services was accompanied by forms of surveillance that laid the foundation for the disruption of families through the child welfare and criminal justice systems. In this concluding chapter, I reflect on the implications of families' experiences for services, policy, and advocacy in the service of cultivating security and equity for marginalized rural families. The lived experiences of the families that participated in this research lay a foundation for practical action to end family homelessness in rural New England, support families' efforts to "make it," and reimagine supportive services for families.

Ending Family Homelessness in Rural New England

Tracing families' experiences over time reveals conditions that either erode or cultivate security following homelessness. In rural New England, the high cost of living and limited housing inventory place families at risk of chronic housing insecurity. Access to affordable housing was the key structural determinant of families' security. Over the course of the research, all the families gained access to subsidized housing for periods of time. Affordable housing facilitated periods of stability for all, ranging from a few months (Abigail) to over a decade (Barbara). Isolation in rural communities, exacerbations of mental illness or substance use, and/or interactions with the child welfare or criminal justice system disrupted periods of stability in affordable housing for Abigail, Tara, Jim, and Hannah. These disruptions offer insights into the need to couple access to affordable housing with a range of other supports for families.

Increasing the inventory of affordable housing in the region is crucial. Vermont has experienced a steady decline in development over the past three decades despite the growth of the state's population (Harrold, 2021). A recent housing needs forecast for the Upper Valley estimates that, by 2030, the region will need to create 10,000 new homes to meet demand—approximately three times more homes than were created in the years 2010 to 2020 (Keys to the Valley, 2022). Efforts to develop housing units need to consider aspects of rural geography, resources, and supports that will enhance families' stability and integration into community life. Developing affordable housing close to town centers in rural communities would help to address many of the challenges that were faced by families in the study, including protecting against loneliness and boredom, lessening transportation challenges, and promoting greater access to health and community resources. There is an opportunity to link the progressive political orientation of Upper Valley communities to practical actions that will increase housing inventory and options for affordable housing in the region.

The development of additional affordable housing in the region faces numerous barriers, including high costs of building materials, workforce shortages in construction, zoning restrictions, lack of infrastructure for higher-density housing in rural communities, lengthy local and state review processes, and poor prioritization of development at the state level (Harrold, 2021). Investments in infrastructure and changes to zoning policies to enable higher-density housing proximate to services and resources will be crucial to increasing opportunities for community members to live and thrive in the Upper Valley. At the community level, not-in-my-backyard (NIMBY) stances toward the development of affordable housing need to be strongly rebuked. Countering stigma associated with poverty through equity-driven policies and community action brings with it the opportunity to disrupt tacit assumptions of the inevitability of homelessness and housing insecurity. Rural New England may be especially well positioned to end homelessness among families. In the 2020 Point-in-Time counts, Vermont reported 124 households with children experiencing homelessness, and New Hampshire reported 219 households with children experiencing homelessness (U.S. Department of Housing and Urban Development, 2021). These numbers, while unacceptably high, are also not overwhelming and should energize efforts to address the housing crisis facing rural New Englanders.

In Vermont, the *Vermont Roadmap to End Homelessness* (Corporation for Supportive Housing, 2016) provides key guidance on policy needs and specific housing approaches, including calling for more supportive housing and more Housing First homeless assistance models (Tsemberis & Eisenberg, 2000). Whereas many housing programs for those mental health or substance use challenges require sobriety and treatment engagement as a condition of gaining access to housing, the Housing First model instead gives immediate access to housing with voluntary connections to mental health and substance use services (Tsemberis, 1999). The Housing First model of providing permanent housing coupled with health, mental health, and other supportive services has been shown to be effective in decreasing homelessness and improving housing stability for populations with physical disabilities, mental illness, and substance use disorders (Peng et al., 2020). A Housing First program in Vermont has an 85% housing retention rate (Stefancic et al., 2013).

The *Vermont Roadmap to End Homelessness* notes that for such approaches to be successful, "an acute shortage of public resources coupled with a well-documented lack of affordable housing across the state must be addressed if homelessness is to end" and further notes that "A significant investment of resources on the part of the State, as well as federal funding, local funding, private philanthropic support and private investments in affordable housing will be required to get the job done" (Corporation for Supportive Housing, 2016, p. 5). Housing advocates assert that solving the region's housing crisis will require the engagement of multiple public and private stakeholders as well as new and innovative approaches given that both the private market and government-run programs "are failing to meet the need in their current form and will continue to fail" (Keys to the Valley, 2022).

As communities and policymakers work toward long-term solutions for affordable housing, the experiences detailed in this book suggest points of departure for creative interim strategies to support families. Doubling up was a key survival strategy used by many families to avoid literal homelessness. Yet these informal arrangements and the stability they offered frayed over time with the pressures of overcrowded spaces, arguments over money, or differences in parenting approaches or housekeeping habits. But what if cohousing approaches could be more intentional and enhanced by supports? Instead of the reinforcement of the New England bootstraps mentality that assumes one family equals one house, supportive cohousing may be a prudent strategy to immediately increase access to housing in the absence of new development. Cohousing may allow families to combine income, lessen social isolation, and enhance parents' ability to balance work and childcare needs. Infused with resources and trauma-informed supports for communication, conflict resolution, problem solving, and parenting, such arrangements could lessen the typical strains on doubling up with others. Supportive cohousing would require formal protections, such as listing multiple names on leases, as well as revision of local ordinances in some communities. While not a one-size-fits-all or necessarily a long-term solution to housing needs in the region, supportive cohousing may be a pragmatic strategy to promote greater security for some families in a context of scarce housing resources and may usefully disrupt the New England bootstrap mentality of self-reliance that undermines and demoralizes many families.

Supporting Families' Efforts to "Make It"

In the context of structural forces that constrain families' ability to "make it" in this rural setting, families engaged in ongoing efforts to live meaningful lives. Daily practices of cooking meals, tending gardens, and keeping house were refashioned as restorative rituals. As families "strive for ordinary," they sought to repair the "moral failures" of homelessness and asserted their "worthiness" (Snell-Rood & Carpenter-Song, 2018) in a cultural setting that valorizes self-reliance. Though families did not use a vocabulary of "hope" to describe these practices, their efforts resonate with Cheryl Mattingly's (2010) conceptualization of hope as situated in everyday actions that offer "an intimation of possibility for a better life even in . . . grim circumstances" (p. 3). Building on families' everyday efforts to cultivate meaningful lives and practical actions to provide for their families, there is an opportunity to amplify these strengths by advocating for practices and policies that address the experiences of fundamental insecurity documented through this ethnographic work.

Families' experiences underscore the need to promote employment opportunities that offer a living wage, regular schedules, and access to healthcare benefits. Parents in the study valued work yet remained unable to "make it" with part-time, low-wage jobs with unpredictable schedules. In this setting, market-rate rents were out of reach for all families in the study. Lacking benefits through employment, parents remained tethered to federal and state benefit programs to ensure continued access to healthcare. In the context of jobs characterized by their insecurity, limited hours, low-wages, and lack of benefits, federal and state benefit programs offered a crucial, though limited, foundation of security through nutritional support, healthcare, and cash benefits. Yet many parents longed to be "off welfare" and to fully support their families' needs through employment.[1]

Families' lived experiences underscored work as a key locus of meaning and structure. This view resonates with evidence from decades of research on supported employment for individuals with mental illnesses (Drake et al., 2012). Expanding evidence-based supported employment programs to people experiencing homelessness may offer opportunities to build collaborative, trusting relationships with an employment specialist (Poremski et al., 2016) who can serve as a guide and advocate to help people find and retain jobs that suit their needs and preferences. Beyond formal services, I also see opportunities to capitalize on strengths of the Upper Valley community to offer greater support of those who have experienced homelessness. The robust volunteer programs within the region's nonprofit sector could be reconfigured so that volunteers are contributing skills specific to their experience, education, and training. For example, retired teachers and professors could translate their years of experience in student advising into serving as mentors; those with legal careers could help individuals to understand their rights and to navigate complex bureaucratic systems; those with policy or community organizing experience could support advocacy efforts for affordable housing, fair wages, access to transportation and childcare.

Limited access to childcare was a key constraint on parents' abilities to work, especially for single mothers with young children. The childcare challenges faced by families in the study mirror the broader reality of the

inadequate childcare infrastructure in the United States (Malik et al., 2018).
The lived realities of working amid such serious constraints strongly counter stigmatizing discourses of those living in poverty being "lazy" or "not
wanting to work."[2] The U.S. is currently at a moment of inflection regarding
economic supports for children and families. The Child Tax Credit implemented in 2021 provided automatic monthly payments to a majority of
working families.[3] This temporary policy, implemented as part of the American Rescue Plan during the COVID-19 pandemic, was intended to reduce
child poverty in the U.S. and also recognizes the high cost of raising children
for both low- and middle-income families. Many advocated for this policy
to become permanent as an investment in children and families. Research
is needed to document both short- and long-term impacts of this policy
change.

Reimagining Supportive Services for Families

Attending closely to families' lived experiences of health and social services
reveals a broad range of perspectives on the nature of problems, with some
ascribing to clinical models of mental illness and substance use and others
deeply skeptical of "psy-" renderings of suffering. Recognizing the diversity
of explanations of and orientations to problems that may be diagnosable as
mental illness or substance use aligns with decades of research in anthropology and cross-cultural psychiatry (Carpenter-Song et al., 2010; Jenkins, 1988;
Jenkins & Barrett, 2004). Beyond diverse explanatory models (Kleinman,
1980), perspectives on specific modalities of treatment also vary. Many participants in the study critiqued narrowly medication-focused treatment,
which is the dominant mode of mental healthcare in many rural areas
(Jenkins & Snell-Rood, 2021). Others were skeptical of therapy, raising concerns about the usefulness of engaging with therapists "who haven't been
through the same stuff." Diverse orientations to treatment were manifest in
the patterns of engagement observed in these families. Some, like Barbara,
did not engage in mental health or substance use treatment during the time
of the research but engaged with other supportive social services "on her
own terms." Others, including Tara and Nancy, were often "going through
the motions" in their interactions with care providers and remained ambivalent and skeptical about the usefulness of services. For Jim and Hannah,
their efforts to engage in a range of services were limited by fragmented

systems of care coupled with stigma and a lack of advocacy that left them "grasping at straws."

These patterns offer insights into missed opportunities within care in rural New England. I argue that most health and social service providers are well-intentioned in their efforts to support the needs of marginalized families. Yet their efforts are constrained by limited resources, fragmented systems, and lack of "structural competence" (Metzl & Hansen, 2014) that produce gaps between the intentions of care and the lived reality of engaging in services. Harms take shape in feelings of judgment, challenges accessing care in rural settings, and a lack of connection with providers.[4] These experiences cast a long shadow and inform expectations of care, rendering many reluctant to seek services. Parents expressed specific reluctance to seek support for mental health and substance use concerns because of fears of child welfare system involvement. Critiquing the "foundational logic" of the child welfare system that emphasizes surveillance and removal of children in marginalized families (Roberts, 2022) may open opportunities to reallocate resources toward services that will keep families together.[5]

Families' orientations to care are not static. By engaging with families over time, I became aware of shifts in their views on and experiences of services. Emblematic of such shifts, as detailed in chapter 6, Nancy grew gradually more open to mental health services over time. Notably, her previously sharp-edged critiques of therapists softened through her children's positive experiences in therapy and her own experiences with particular providers. Just as negative experiences inform expectations for care, so, too, do positive ones. Families' lived experiences of care—positive and negative—point to possibilities for reimagining supportive services for those living with the multiple burdens of poverty, mental illness, and substance use in rural settings. As I noted in chapter 1, my articulation of strategies is oriented by a model of accompaniment in which "Interventions are not to be proposed 'from the outside,' but determined with participants, alongside, through critical dialogue and reflection" (Watkins, 2015, p. 329).

Health and social services need to meaningfully attend to the lived realities of surviving in poverty. This includes deepening awareness of the social responses and cultural orientations to poverty and homelessness. In rural New England, the valorization of self-reliance shapes the meanings and experiences of vulnerability. Families were subject to harsh forms of social exclusion and internalized shame associated with poverty in this setting. The New England bootstrap mentality may discourage many from seeking help, shaping if and how people engage with health and social service providers. Moreover, the pervasive stigma endured by families may further reinforce expectations and fears of being judged by others, including by care providers. In this context, seeking support requires the strength to go against expectations of self-reliance and the courage to risk encountering stigma and judgment. Cultivating an ethos within systems of care that actively acknowledges efforts to engage in supportive services as demonstrations of strength and courage may offer a point of departure for building more trusting relationships. As Mary Watkins (2015) advocates, "The resilience of those accompanied and their own cultural resources for understanding and healing need to be cherished and supported, not usurped" (p. 329). Orienting individuals to care, including acknowledging past harms and honest discussions of the usefulness and limitations of specific therapeutic modalities, is foundational to the work of care with marginalized families.

Reimagining supportive services will require redesigning systems and reforming structures that amplify vulnerabilities and reinforce inequities. Health and social service providers need training in the social determinants of health and trauma-informed care. The "shattering" of families detailed in chapter 5 compels examination of the potentially devastating unintended consequences of care that can result from frayed, fragmented, and underfunded systems. Although families relied on supportive services to meet their survival needs, engagement in health and social services entails exposure as those experiencing homelessness "parent in public" (Friedman, 2000). Parents were keenly aware of how being poor and experiencing mental health or substance use challenges could raise questions about their fitness as parents. Despite the prominence and wide acceptance of explanatory models of mental illness and addiction as brain disorders, parents struggling with these conditions remained deeply stigmatized (cf. Jenkins & Carpenter-Song, 2005). With respect to mental illness, "The assumption by the lay public and even seasoned clinicians is that women with mental illness either don't become mothers or are incapable of parenting their children" (Benders-Hadi & Barber, 2014, p. ix). By contrast, research with parents who have mental illnesses demonstrates that parenting is a core locus of meaning (Carpenter-Song et al., 2014; Mowbray, Oyserman, & Ross, 1995) and a foundational resource for recovery (Nicholson et al., 1998). Treatment approaches such as the family recovery model (Nicholson, 2014) offer a promising vision of services oriented by partnering with families "to acknowledge the strengths and resources women bring to the challenges of mothering, build on these to achieve their goals, facilitate access to essential environmental resources and supports, and enhance positive elements of recovery in the context of family life" (p. 8). For parents with substance use disorders, model approaches also exist that support "policies based on prevention and family preservation" rather than "traditions of rescue and punishment" (Carten, 1996, p. 222).[6]

Recovery in the Context of Homelessness

As an anthropologist of mental health, I have attended closely to the meanings and experiences of psychiatric recovery throughout my career (Carpenter-Song et al., 2012; Carpenter-Song et al., 2014; Jenkins & Carpenter-Song, 2005). The paradigmatic shift toward recovery in the context of mental health upended expectations of the inevitability of serious mental illnesses as invariably degenerative diseases (Jenkins & Carpenter-Song, 2005). As clinical psychologist and mental health advocate Patricia Deegan powerfully asserts, "We are a conspiracy of hope and we are pressing back against the strong tide of oppression. . . . people who have been diagnosed with mental illnesses are not things, not objects to be acted upon, are not animals or subhuman lifeforms. . . . Our lives are precious and are of infinite value" (1987, p. 2). What if we entered a similar conspiracy of hope with those enduring homelessness and housing insecurity? Cheryl Mattingly (2010) reminds us that

> Things can seem hopeless from a theoretical perspective if one isn't careful . . . and sees only the overwhelming, apparently overdetermining social structures that seem to ensure the reproduction of dramatic inequalities. It would be foolhardy, especially in this particular historical period, to ignore the devastating machinery, both global and national, that perpetuates chilling economic and political inequities. But it is equally foolhardy to neglect the ways even those who are most oppressed locate and cultivate "resources of hope" [Williams, 1989] that offer reasons to live and to act. (p. 24)

With the possibility of recovery as an orienting principle, it becomes crucial to recognize the constellation of personal effort (Substance Abuse and Mental Health Services Administration, 2004), social context (Mezzina et al., 2006; Myers, 2015), and structures (Jenkins & Csordas, 2020) that must be brought to bear in cultivating meaningful recovery for those living in poverty and struggling with mental health and substance use challenges. Janis Jenkins and Thomas Csordas (2020) articulate this nexus of possibility in this way:

> It is clear that subjective possibilities of hope and transformation—when marked by the impress of social extremity—are largely contingent on the availability of institutional-structural pathways and environments to take care of lives, establish well-being, achieve equity, and ensure equanimity. (p. 245)

As anthropologists, we situate our work at the intersection of the empirical and the space of imagination. Intimate forms of ethnography allow us to see beauty in the quotidian and strength in the struggle. We document, through our intensive modes of engagement and bearing witness, what is and also wonder at what could be. In this work, long-term participation with families has illuminated both the catalysts of disruption and of possibility. *Things could have been otherwise.* With this view, we turn toward the suffering not through the spectral gaze of the academic voyeur[7] but instead with the ever-incisive eye of solidarity. Tragic outcomes become an invitation into "angry indignation" (Deegan, 1993, p. 9) and demand that we ask: *How could this have ended differently for this family?* Those who moved toward greater security over time compel the question: *How can more families have access to structural resources and supports that can amplify their strengths?*

As such, I choose to end this book not with a statement but with a question. Whether you are reading this as a student, a care provider, a community member, or someone with lived experience, I ask: *What can you do to create interactions and environments that destabilize stigma, promote compassion, and advocate for equity?*

Epilogue: Notes from the Pandemic

The experiences detailed in this book stretch back more than decade. I began this work in the shadow of the Great Recession of 2008 and wrote most of this book during 2020 and 2021 amid the COVID-19 pandemic. These experiential bookends each held and continue to hold deep implications for housing and health in the region.

Early spring is always a time of anticipation in this part of Northern New England—a vigil of attunement to the gradual lengthening of days, the return of birdsong, and the yielding of snow to mud to delicate green blades. These usual rhythms were layered with a darker sort of anticipation as we all witnessed scenes of New York transformed into the largest global outbreak of COVID-19 in the spring of 2020. Keenly aware of our shared borders with New York State and Massachusetts, the region braced for what seemed to be an inevitable surge of COVID cases. Yet, as spring turned to summer in 2020, case counts remained low in the region, sparing rural communities and health systems. Unlike in highly populated U.S. settings in which the pandemic announced itself daily—in the wail of sirens, the presence of refrigerated trailers serving as roadside morgues, and collective rituals of gratitude for healthcare workers—in Northern New England the morbidity and mortality of the pandemic were less visible for most people through the fall of 2020. Instead, in rural Vermont and New Hampshire, the realities of the pandemic were manifest primarily in social and economic impacts.

In the small towns and villages where "everyone knows everyone," there was an awareness of shared vulnerability—of the elderly; of community members who had recently lost jobs; of schoolchildren thrust into remote learning and newly untethered from supports; of those with disabilities and chronic illnesses; and of those experiencing homelessness, mental illness, or substance use. For the families whose experiences are detailed in this book, the pandemic profoundly changed their everyday lives. Like so many workers deemed "essential," Barbara continued her work at a local market amid a swirl of fear, uncertainty, and new protocols. With continued access to affordable housing and stable (though challenging) employment, Barbara has maintained her family's housing. For Nancy, as for many women in the United States, the abrupt closing of schools and transitioning to remote learning for schoolchildren meant that she could no longer work outside the home. Unemployed for over 18 months, Nancy relied on governmental supports through the American Rescue Plan to maintain her family's access to housing, nutrition, and other basic needs. In the fall of 2021, schools fully reopened, and Nancy interviewed for jobs and re-entered the workforce.

In rural New England, as elsewhere in the country, the pandemic laid bare longstanding inequalities. Yet early in the response to the pandemic, rural communities and health systems mobilized rapidly to meet the needs of medically and socially vulnerable rural residents (Sosin & Carpenter-Song, 2020). Rural clinics and hospitals worked to identify high-risk patients and dispatched community health workers to provide support. School districts repurposed bus routes to deliver meals to children reliant on school-based nutrition programs. Village committees delivered groceries and medicines to isolated elders and meals to families left newly unemployed. In Vermont, concerns over the high risk of infection in congregate shelter settings led to the expansion of eligibility for motel vouchers to house those at risk of homelessness, the enactment of an eviction moratorium, and rent relief for landlords (Sosin et al., 2021). At community and policy levels, there was a prioritization of those most at risk of contracting severe illness from COVID-19 as well as those bearing the impact of economic losses and social isolation.

The actions taken during the earliest days of the pandemic illuminate what is possible when communities, institutions, and policies align to meet the needs of medically vulnerable and marginalized rural residents. These efforts also suggest a tempering of the New England bootstrap mentality through collective actions to protect rural residents and communities. Now, as the region moves beyond the pandemic crisis response, there is a critical opportunity to extend the community strengths, energy, and political will to continue to prioritize the needs of marginalized rural New Englanders and address longstanding health equity challenges in the region.

Appendix: Family Housing Trajectories

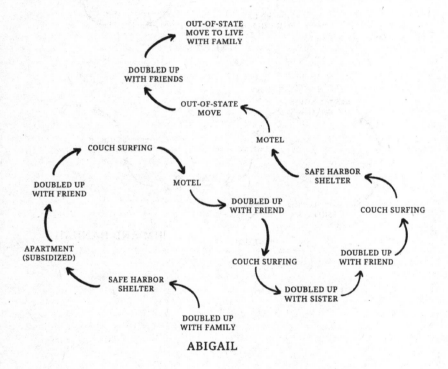

ABIGAIL

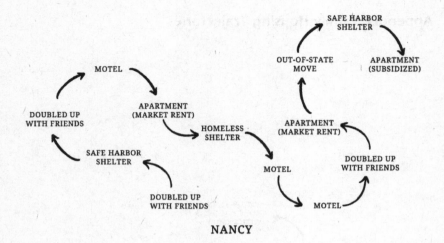

NANCY

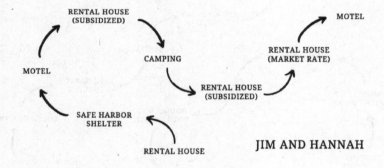

JIM AND HANNAH

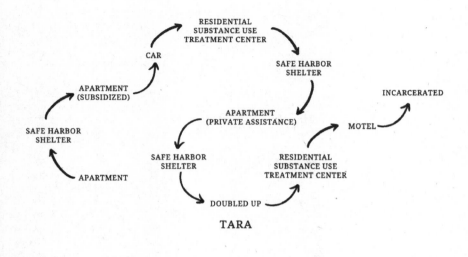

TARA

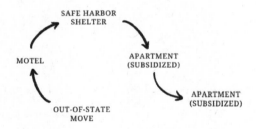

BARBARA

Notes

Chapter 1

1. As an example, debates over affordable housing have unfolded over two decades in Norwich, Vermont—a small town (population 3,353) with a median household income of $117,069 in 2020, making it one of the wealthiest towns in the state (and, indeed, the United States). A private nonprofit group, Norwich Affordable Housing Inc., reignited this debate in calling for the construction of "mixed income" housing targeted at bringing in families earning about $45,000 a year. This project was met with fierce objection by many town residents—despite the town's progressive reputation. The nonprofit group has since disbanded.

2. A notable exception is the work of sociologist Janet Fitchen (1991, 1992) in upstate New York in the 1990s.

3. This question would be prompted by annual renewals of institutional review boards (IRBs) and in anticipation of the ending of grants.

4. During this time, I was not able to afford a local apartment while still based out of state. For housing arrangements, I leaned on the generosity of friends and, through word of mouth, eventually found space in a rooming house frequented by traveling nurses. Notably, this arrangement was possible because of my status as an adult with no children in the early years of the research.

5. My own life experiences have ranged across different circumstances. As I was growing up, my parents struggled financially, and I was aware of scarcity and struggle. Yet I do not bring lived experience of deep poverty or homelessness, and I acknowledge the privilege of having had parents who deeply valued and supported education. But these varying life experiences have facilitated my capacities to move across and between contexts and circumstances—a foundational skill for an anthropologist.

6. Families received $50 per month regardless of the number of research contacts during that time. They were not compensated on a per-visit basis. This design was meant to limit the possibility of the compensation being coercive.

7. I situate this work as engaged, action-oriented research.

8. Visits occurred at least monthly from 2009 to 2012 and bimonthly thereafter. Visits often occurred more frequently, and all participants maintained regular contact with me by text message and telephone between visits. All five families participated from 2009 to 2014. By 2015, two families stopped engaging in the study. From 2016 to the present, two families have continued to engage regularly.

9. This average is brought down substantially from market-rate rents in the region due to the fact that some families in the study received housing subsidies, which capped their out-of-pocket expenses.

10. One mother identified her child as multiethnic.

Chapter 2

1. There are many definitions of *rural*. In this study, I defined *rural* in accordance with the U.S. Department of Agriculture Economic Research Service. The research was conducted in Windsor County, Vermont; Orange County, Vermont; and Grafton County, New Hampshire. All three counties are designated as nonmetropolitan areas.

   The population densities of the towns where participants resided during the study ranged from 17.3 persons per square mile (Vershire, VT) to 326.2 persons per square mile (Lebanon, NH) (Vermont State Government, 2013; New Hampshire Economic & Labor Market Information Bureau, 2013). In less technical terms, participants described living in "small towns" and "villages" or, in more remote locations, "the middle of nowhere."

2. Awareness of housing as a challenge facing the region has grown during the time of the study. While there is increased awareness and growing advocacy around housing, this has not yet translated into substantial changes in the landscape of affordable housing in the region.

3. From January 2020 to June 2020, the number of people staying in state-funded housing increased from 1,100 to 2,000 due to COVID-19-related financial burdens (Elletson, 2020).

4. Images of the "other America" from the 1960s War on Poverty (Harrington, 1962; Johnson, 1964) are emblematic of the cultural imagination surrounding rural poverty. Similar depictions exist in contemporary coverage of the opioid epidemic in rural areas.

5. As noted in chapter 1, efforts to develop affordable housing have met resistance among residents in the region. Other barriers specific to the development of higher density include infrastructural constraints common to rural areas, such as a lack of sewer lines.

6. At one point during the study, I observed an exception to this pattern. Three families in one pod became quite close and interacted regularly. They frequently played card games together and often cooked a shared meal. One of the three families

included an older woman who quickly took on the role of pod grandmother. Having multiple generations present may have facilitated stronger connections.

7. Over the course of the research, Jim and Hannah were engaged in a protracted custody case with the state of Vermont following the placement of their four children in state custody in the fall of 2009. Stable housing was a condition of their reunification. As is examined in detail in chapter 5, despite achieving this goal, their parental rights were ultimately terminated.

8. Although today the expression "pulling yourself up by your bootstraps" is used to idealize the American cultural narrative of the self-made man and signify the expectation that one ought to be self-reliant, early uses of this expression were instead intended to express efforts to do something absurd or impossible, according to linguistic research by Benjamin Zimmer (Zimmer, 2005; see also Bologna, 2018).

Chapter 4

1. Community-based mental health services such as assertive community treatment (ACT) were developed in the context of deinstitutionalization in the United States in the 1960s and 1970s. These models of care emphasized providing a range of supports to people in the community and "acknowledged people's broad needs for simple survival in the post-asylum era. Often poor, unemployed, and marginalized, this group faced not only the fragmented mental health system but also the dispersal (or nonexistence) of all the other services that once came bundled togher in the state hospital" (Brodwin, 2013, p. 36). Yet, as Paul Brodwin (2013) compellingly argues in his ethnography of front-line clinicians, there is a chasm between a promise of such models and the reality of care provided by lower-level mental health professionals. He describes the "perverse logic" of public services for those with mental illness: "Clinicians with the least training, lowest pay, and lease control over their work inherit responsibility for the most disabled and marginalized individuals" (Brodwin, 2013, p. 3).

Street psychiatry aims to bring mental health and substance use treatment directly to individuals experiencing unsheltered homelessness in recognition of the significant barriers to access to healthcare and the high needs of this population (Christensen, 2009; Lam & Rosenheck, 1999).

Chapter 5

1. One family requested that I testify in their termination of parental rights (TPR) hearing. After much reflection, I declined, explaining my concern that the settings and interactions that I had observed in the course of my time with the family might not be viewed favorably and that my involvement might be more harmful than helpful.

2. I use the term "self" intentionally (1) to evoke Irving Hallowell's (1955) sense of the experiencing subject, (2) to reflect the experience-near vocabulary within the settings in

which I work, and (3) to facilitate engagement with longstanding inquiries into "self" within psychological anthropology. Questioning cultural assumptions regarding the unitary and stable self has been fundamental to the field of psychological anthropology.

3. Psychological anthropologists have called attention to our capacity for shifting and "multiple selves" (Ochs & Capps, 1996). Yet some transformations of self-experience seem to exceed this malleability. The parents described in this chapter experience fundamental changes in their identities and in their orientations to time and space. Parents and children offer a paradigmatic site for examining intersubjectivity, underscoring the relational constitution of the self (Csordas, 1994) and moral experience—the "I" connected inextricably to the "we" (Mattingly, 2014; Zigon, 2014). The tragic outcomes detailed in this chapter underscore the inherent vulnerability and risk entailed in the relational constitution of subjects (Zigon & Throop, 2014).

4. Tara's rent was subsidized and thus capped at 30% of her income.

5. They both had adult children from previous relationships and had four younger children together.

6. Annette Appell (1998) argues that the child welfare system focuses on "fixing" women: "mothers' conduct, psychological makeup, compliance, and drug and alcohol use [become] the focus. If the mothers are the problem, then it is they who must be fixed. To be fixed, however, they must become different women. From this perspective, failure is usually a foregone conclusion" (p. 376).

7. Jarrett Zigon and C. Jason Throop (2014) claim that a significant aspect of moral experience lies in the care of relations: "ethical practices are not for the sake of the Other but rather ultimately work to maintain, repair, or make new relations that ultimately results in the maintenance, repair, or making anew of both oneself and all those other constituted through the relationship cared for" (p. 9). This chapter documents the devastating consequences that occur when the possibilities for caring for those relations are permanently severed by state intervention.

8. For example, when Tara asked for help in the substance-abuse treatment facility, this request was recast as an inability to parent her children. Tara lost her subsidized housing when her kids were taken into state custody, yet a condition of reunification was that she would secure housing. Jim and Hannah reported that their lawyer stated during a court hearing, "I've never seen DCF [Department of Children and Families] be this vindictive with a family!"

Chapter 6

1. After living in the same place for 12 months with a voucher, the voucher holder can change properties or even move to a different state (Miller, 2020).

2. Nancy had already reached her five-year limit on receiving Temporary Aid to Needy Families (TANF), but recent pandemic-specific policy revisions allowed her to receive cash benefits during the pandemic.

Chapter 7

1. Critiques of an overemphasis on paid work in the context of psychiatric recovery (Myers, 2015) serve as a reminder of the importance of recognizing—and cultivating—many opportunities for creating meaningful lives.

2. The long shadow of Ronald Reagan's 1976 "welfare queen" speech is evident in current debates regarding the serious labor shortages in the United States in the wake of the COVID-19 pandemic. Whereas conservative discourse posits that these labor shortages reflect a broad preference for not working, progressives argue instead that shortages are reflective of growing resistance toward untenable working conditions, particularly in low-wage, service-sector jobs.

3. Under the Biden administration in 2021, the annual Child Tax Credit was increased from $2,000 per child to $3,000 (for children older than six) and $3,600 (for children younger than six). Families receive the full credit if they earn up to $150,000 for a two-parent household or $112,500 for a family with a single parent (White House, n.d.).

4. The families in this research faced many challenges, but they did not experience institutional racism given that all self-identified as White. Because homelessness disproportionately impacts Black and indigenous populations in the United States (Henry, 2020), in other geographic settings it is likely that families experiencing homelessness would also be subject to institutional racism in the context of health and social services.

5. Dorothy Roberts (2021) notes that the federal government devoted $8.6 billion to maintaining children in foster care in 2019. This is more than 10 times the amount allocated to supportive services aimed at keeping families together (Roberts 2021, p. 68).

6. Alma Carten (1996) describes the Family Rehabilitation Program implemented in New York City in response to significant increases in foster care caseloads in the context of substance abuse. The program recognized the systemic inequities that placed poor women of color at increased risk of child welfare system involvement. Specific to the context of this research, the Moms in Recovery program at Dartmouth Hitchcock Medical Center provides services to pregnant and parenting women with substance use disorders. The program was started in 2013 through a collaboration between the hospital's departments of psychiatry and obstetrics and gynecology. The program aims to provide holistic care by attending to the medical and social needs of women in recovery (Dartmouth Hitchcock Medical Center and Clinics, n.d.).

7. Joel Robbins (2013) has critiqued anthropological engagements with suffering as reproducing the "savage slot" in anthropology.

References

Adoption and Safe Families Act, Pub. L. 105-89, 111 Stat. 2115 (1997). https://www
.gpo.gov/fdsys/pkg/PLAW-105publ89/pdf/PLAW-105publ89.pdf

Ali, M. M., Teich, J. L., & Mutter, R. (2015). The role of perceived need and health insurance in substance use treatment: Implications for the Affordable Care Act. *Journal of Substance Abuse Treatment, 54*, 14.

Allegretto, S., Doussard, M., Graham-Squire, D., Jacobs, K., Thompson, D., & Thompson, J. (2013). *Fast food, poverty wages: The public cost of low-wage jobs in the fast-food industry.* University of California, Berkeley, Center for Labor Research and Education and the University of Illinois at Urbana-Champaign Department of Urban & Regional Planning. laborcenter.berkeley.edu/pdf/2013/fast_food_poverty_wages.pdf

Amore, K., Baker, M., & Howden-Chapman, P. (2011). The ETHOS definition and classification of homelessness: An analysis. *European Journal of Homelessness, 5*(2), 19–37.

Annie E. Casey Foundation. (2017). KIDS COUNT Data Center. Retrieved August 31, 2017, from http://datacenter.kidscount.org/

Appell, A. R. (1998). On fixing "bad" mothers and saving their children. In M. Ladd-Taylor & L. Umansky, *"Bad" mothers: The politics of blame in twentieth-century America* (pp. 356–380). New York University Press.

Barrow, S. M., & Laborde, N. D. (2008). Invisible mothers: Parenting by homeless women separated from their children. *Gender Issues, 25*, 157–172.

Barrow, S. M., & Lawinski, T. (2009). Contexts of mother-child separations in homeless families. *Analyses of Social Issues and Public Policy, 9*(1), 157–176.

Bassuk, E. (1993). "Homeless women: Economic and Social Issues—Introduction." *American Journal of Orthopsychiatry, 63*, 337–339.

Bech, T. (2015). Testimony on S. 9 to members of the (Vermont) House Human Services Committee, March 19. Vermont Parent Representation Center, Inc.

Benders-Hadi, N., & Barber, M. E. (Eds.). (2014). *Motherhood, mental illness and recovery: Stories of hope.* Springer.

Biederman, D. J., & Lindsey, E. W. (2014). Promising research and methodological approaches for health behavior research with homeless persons. *Journal of Social Distress and the Homeless, 23*(2), 105–108.

Biehl, J. (2005). *Vita: Life in a zone of social abandonment.* University of California Press.

Biehl, J., Good, B. J., & Kleinman, A. (Eds.). (2007). *Subjectivity: Ethnographic investigations.* University of California Press.

Bologna, C. (2018, August 9). "Why the phrase 'pull yourself up by your bootstraps' is nonsense." *Huffpost.* https://www.huffpost.com/entry/pull-yourself-up-by-your-bootstraps-nonsense_n_5b1ed024e4b0bbb7a0e037d4

Braun, V., & Clarke, V. (2006). Using thematic analysis in psychology. *Qualitative Research in Psychology, 3*(2), 77–101.

Braveman, P., & Gottlieb, L. (2014). The social determinants of health: It's time to consider the causes of the causes. *Public Health Reports, 129*(Suppl. 2), 19–31.

Brodwin, P. (2013). *Everyday ethics: Voices from the front line of community psychiatry.* University of California Press.

Bruner, E. M. (1986). Experience and its expressions. In V. W. Turner & E. M. Bruner (Eds.), *The anthropology of experience* (pp. 3–30). University of Illinois Press.

Buckner, J. C., Bassuk, E. L., & Zima, B. T. (1993). Mental health issues affecting homeless women: Implications for intervention. *American Journal of Orthopsychiatry, 63*(3), 385–399.

Bullon, A., Good, M. J. D., & Carpenter-Song, E. (2011). Paper life: Documentation practices in the care of minority and low-income patients. In M. J. DelVecchio Good, S. S. Willen, S. D. Hannah, K. Vickery, & L. T. Park (Eds.), *Shattering culture: American medicine responds to cultural diversity* (pp. 200–216). Russell Sage Foundation.

Butler, S. S. (1997). Homelessness among AFDC families in a rural state: It is bound to get worse. *Affilia, 12,* 427–451.

Carpenter-Song, E. (2009a). Caught in the psychiatric net: Meanings and experiences of ADHD, pediatric bipolar disorder and mental health treatment among a diverse group of families in the United States. *Culture, Medicine and Psychiatry, 33*(1), 61–85.

Carpenter-Song, E. (2009b). Children's sense of self in relation to clinical processes: Portraits of pharmaceutical transformation. *Ethos, 37*(3), 257–281.

Carpenter-Song, E. (2011). Recognition in clinical relationships. In M.-J. DelVecchio Good, S. S. Willen, S. D. Hannah, K. Vickery, & L. T. Park (Eds.), *Shattering culture: American medicine responds to cultural diversity* (pp. 168–183). Russell Sage Foundation.

Carpenter-Song, E., Chu, E., Drake, R. E., Ritsema, M., Smith, B., & Alverson, H. (2010). Ethno-cultural variations in the experience and meaning of mental illness and treatment: Implications for access and utilization. *Transcultural Psychiatry, 47*(2), 224–251.

Carpenter-Song, E., Ferron, J., & Kobylenski, S. (2016). Social exclusion and survival for families facing homelessness in rural New England. *Journal of Social Distress and the Homeless, 25*(1), 41–52.

Carpenter-Song, E., Hipolito, M., & Whitley, R. (2012). "Right here is an oasis": How "recovery communities" contribute to recovery for people with serious mental illnesses. *Psychiatric Rehabilitation Journal, 35*(6), 435–440.

Carpenter-Song, E., Holcombe, B., Torrey, J., Hipolito, M., & Peterson, L. (2014). Recovery in a family context: Experiences of mothers with serious mental illnesses. *Psychiatric Rehabilitation Journal, 37*(3), 162–169.

Carpenter-Song, E. A., Schwallie, M. N., & Longhofer, J. (2007). Cultural competence reexamined: Critique and directions for the future. *Psychiatric Services, 58*(10), 1362–1365.

Carten, A. J. (1996). Mothers in recovery: Rebuilding families in the aftermath of addiction. *Social Work, 41*(2), 214–223.

Case, A., & Deaton, A. (2020). *Deaths of despair and the future of capitalism.* Princeton University Press.

Center on Budget and Policy Priorities. (2019). Vermont Federal Rental Assistance Fact Sheet. Federal Rental Assistance Fact Sheets. Retrieved October 28, 2020, from https://www.cbpp.org/research/housing/federal-rental-assistance-fact-sheets#VT

Christensen, R. C. (2009). Psychiatric street outreach to homeless people: Fostering relationship, reconnection, and recovery. *Journal of Health Care for the Poor and Underserved, 20*(4), 1036–1040.

Cloke, P., Milbourne, P., & Widdowfield, R. (2000). Homelessness and rurality: "Out-of-place" in purified space? *Environment and Planning D: Society and Space, 18*(6), 715–735.

Cloke, P., Milbourne, P., & Widdowfield, R. (2003). The complex mobilities of homeless people in rural England. *Geoforum, 34*(1), 21–35.

Corporation for Supportive Housing (CSH). (2016). *Vermont roadmap to end homelessness.* Retrieved October 12, 2022, from https://vhcb.org/sites/default/files/pdfs/pubs/VT-Roadmap-to-End-Homelessness-Final-Report-2016-12-20.pdf

Cosgrove, L., & Flynn, C. (2005). Marginalized mothers: Parenting without a home. *Analyses of Social Issues and Public Policy, 5*, 127–143.

Craft-Rosenberg, M., Powell, S. R., Culp, K., & Iowa Homeless Research Team. (2000). Health status and resources of rural homeless women and children. *Western Journal of Nursing Research, 22*(8), 863–878.

Crist, L., & Bech, T. (2018). Bending the curve to improve our child protection system: A multiyear analysis of Vermont's Child Protection System and recommendation for improvement. Vermont Parent Representation Center, Inc. https://vtprc.org/wp-content/uploads/2018/11/BTC-11-09-18-FINAL.pdf

Csordas, T. J. (1994). *The sacred self: A cultural phenomenology of charismatic healing*. University of California Press.

Dartmouth Hitchcock Medical Center and Clinics. (n.d.). Moms in recovery. Dartmouth Health. http://dartmouth-hitchcock.org/psychiatry/moms-recovery

Das, V., & Kleinman, A. (2001). *Remaking a world: Violence, social suffering, and recovery*. University of California Press.

Deegan, P. (1987). *Recovery, rehabilitation and the conspiracy of hope*. Address to the National Empowerment Center. Retrieved September 13, 2021, from https://citeseerx.ist.psu.edu/viewdoc/download?doi=10.1.1.730.7090&rep=rep1&type=pdf

Deegan, P. E. (1993). Recovering our sense of value after being labeled mentally ill. *Journal of Psychosocial Nursing and Mental Health Services, 31*(4), 7–11.

Desmond, M. (2016). *Evicted: Poverty and profit in the American city*. Broadway Books.

Dew, B., Elifson, K., & Dozier, M. 2007. Social and environmental factors and their influence on drug use vulnerability and resiliency in rural populations. *Journal of Rural Health, 23*, 16–21.

Doyle, J. J. 2007. Child protection and child outcomes: Measuring the effects of foster care. *American Economic Review, 97*(5), 1583–1610.

Drake, R. E., Bond, G. R., & Becker, D. R. (2012). *Individual placement and support: An evidence-based approach to supported employment*. Oxford University Press.

Dunlap, K. M., & Fogel, S. J. (1998). A preliminary analysis of research on recovery from homelessness. *Journal of Social Distress and the Homeless, 7*(3), 175–188.

Elletson, G. (2020, June 7). After COVID-19 crisis, where will homeless Vermonters go? *VT Digger*. https://vtdigger.org/2020/06/go/07/after-covid-19-crisis-where-will-homeless-vermonters-go/

Emerson, R. M., Fretz, R. I., & Shaw, L. L. (2011). *Writing ethnographic fieldnotes*. University of Chicago Press.

Engel, G. L. (1977). The need for a new medical model: a challenge for biomedicine. *Science, 196*(4286), 129–136.

Farmer, P. (1996). On suffering and structural violence: A view from below. *Daedalus, 125*(1), 261–283.

Farmer, P. (2013). *To repair the world: Paul Farmer speaks to the next generation*. University of California Press.

Federal Reserve. (2019, May). *Report on the economic well-being of U.S. households in 2018.* https://www.federalreserve.gov/publications/2019-economic-well-being-of-us -households-in-2018-dealing-with-unexpected-expenses.htm

First, R. J., Rife, J. C., & Toomey, B. G. (1994). Homelessness in rural areas: Causes, patterns, and trends. *Social Work, 39,* 97–108.

Fitchen, J. (1991). Homelessness in rural places: Perspectives from upstate New York. *Urban Anthropology, 20*(2), 177–210.

Fitchen, J. (1992). On the edge of homelessness: Rural poverty and housing insecurity. *Rural Sociology, 57*(2), 173–193.

Fong, K. (2017). Child welfare involvement and contexts of poverty: The role of parental adversities, social networks, and social services. *Child and Youth Services Review, 72,* 5–13.

Foucault, M. (1994). *The birth of the clinic: An archaelogy of medical perception.* Vintage Books.

Fox, J., Merwin, E., & Blank, M. (1995). De facto mental health services in the rural south. *Journal of Health Care for the Poor and Underserved, 6*(4), 434–468.

Friedman, D. H. (2000). *Parenting in public: Family shelter and public assistance.* Columbia University Press.

Garcia, A. (2008). The elegaic addict: History, chronicity, and the melancholic subject. *Cultural Anthropology, 23*(4), 718–746.

Good, B. (1994). *Medicine, rationality, and experience: An anthropological perspective.* Cambridge University Press.

Good, M. D. (1995). *American medicine: The quest for competence.* University of California Press.

Good, M. D., James, C., Good, B. J., & Becker, A. E. (2005). The culture of medicine and racial, ethnic, and class disparities in healthcare. In M. Romero & E. Margolis (Eds.), *The Blackwell companion to social inequalities* (pp. 396–423). Blackwell.

Haas, B. (2017). Citizens-in-waiting, deportees-in-waiting: Power, temporality, and suffering in the U.S. asylum system. *Ethos, 45*(1), 75–97.

Hallowell, I. (1955). *Culture and experience.* University of Pennsylvania Press.

Hampton, R. L., & Newberger, E. H. (1985). Child abuse incidence and reporting by hospitals: Significance of severity, class, and race. *American Journal of Public Health, 75*(1), 56–60.

Hansen, H. (2019). Substance-induced psychosis: Clinical-racial subjectivities and capital in diagnostic apartheid. *Ethos, 47*(1), 73–88.

Hansen, H., Braslow, J., & Rohrbaugh, R. M. (2018). From cultural to structural competency: Training psychiatry residents to act on social determinants of health and institutional racism. *JAMA Psychiatry, 75*(2), 117–118.

Harrington, M. (1962). *The other America: Poverty in the United States*. Touchstone.

Harris, M. E., & Fallot, R. D. (2001). *Using trauma theory to design service systems*. Jossey-Bass/Wiley.

Harrold, B. (2021). *Affordable housing: Barriers and incentives in Vermont towns*. Vermont Housing Finance Agency Report. https://vhfa.org/sites/default/files/publications/Affordable_housing_barriers_VT_towns.pdf

Hauenstein, E. J., & Peddada, S. D. (2007). Prevalence of major depressive episodes in rural women using primary care. *Journal of Health Care for the Poor and Underserved, 18*(1), 185–202.

Henry, M., et al. (2020). *The 2020 annual homeless assessment report (AHAR) to Congress*. U.S. Department of Housing and Urban Development, Office of Community Planning and Development. https://www.huduser.gov/portal/sites/default/files/pdf/2020-AHAR-Part-1.pdf

Hirsch, J. K., & Cukrowicz, K. C. (2014). Suicide in rural areas: An updated review of the literature. *Journal of Rural Mental Health, 38*(2), 65–78.

Hochschild, A. R. (2016). *Strangers in their own land: Anger and mourning on the American right*. New Press.

Hojat, M., Mangione, S., Nasca, T. J., Rattner, S., Erdmann, J. B., Gonnella, J. S., & Magee, M. 2004. An empirical study of decline in empathy in medical school. *Medical Education, 38*(9), 934–941.

Hongoltz-Hetling, M. (2017, March 3). State's attorney puts White River Junction's Shady Lawn Motel on notice. *Valley News*. https://www.vnews.com/Shady-Lawn-Motel-focus-of-officials-8419060

hooks, b. (2000). *Where we stand: Class matters*. Routledge.

Hopper, K. (1991) Homelessness old and new: The matter of definition. *Housing Policy Debate, 2*(3), 755–813.

Hopper, K. (2003). *Reckoning with homelessness*. Cornell University Press.

Hopper, K. (2006). Redistribution and its discontents: On the prospects of committed work in public mental health and like settings. *Human Organization, 65*(2), 218–226.

Jackson, M. (2013). *Lifeworlds: Essays in existential anthropology*. University of Chicago Press.

Jenkins, J. H. (1988). Conceptions of schizophrenia as a problem of nerves: A cross-cultural comparison of Mexican-Americans and Anglo-Americans. *Social Science & Medicine, 26*(12), 1233–1243.

Jenkins, J. H. (1991). The state construction of affect: Political ethos and mental health among Salvadoran refugees. *Culture Medicine and Psychiatry, 15,* 139–165.

Jenkins, J. H. (1997). Subjective perception of persistent schizophrenia among U.S. Latinos and Euro-Americans. *British Journal of Psychiatry, 171*(1), 20–25.

Jenkins, J. H. (2015a). *Extraordinary conditions: Culture and experience in mental illness.* University of California Press.

Jenkins, J. H. (2015b). Straining psychic and social sinew: Trauma among adolescent psychiatric patients in New Mexico. *Medical Anthropology Quarterly, 29*(1), 42–60.

Jenkins, J. H., & Barrett, R. J. (Eds.). (2004). *Schizophrenia, culture, and subjectivity: The edge of experience.* Cambridge University Press.

Jenkins, J. H., & Carpenter-Song, E. (2005). The new paradigm of recovery from schizophrenia: Cultural conundrums of improvement without cure. *Culture, Medicine and Psychiatry, 29*(4), 379–413.

Jenkins, J. H., & Csordas, T. (2020). *Troubled in the land of enchantment: Experience of psychiatric treatment.* University of California Press.

Jenkins, R., & Snell-Rood, C. (2021). Rural perspectives challenging pharmacotherapy. *Journal of Behavioral Health Services & Research, 48*(1), 112–119.

Johnson, L. B. (1964, January 8). The war on poverty. First State of the Union Address. Washington, DC.

Jonson-Reid, M., Drake, B., & Kohl, P. L. (2009). Is the overrepresentation of the poor in child welfare caseloads due to bias or need? *Children and Youth Services Review, 31*(3), 422–427.

Kay, J. B. (2009). Representing parents with disabilities in child protection proceedings. *Michigan Child Welfare Law Journal, 13*(1), 28–36.

Kelly, A. (2014, September 28). The experts the Ebola virus may need: anthropologists [radio broadcast]. National Public Radio. Retrieved October 4, 2022, from https://www.npr.org/sections/goatsandsoda/2014/09/28/351845664/the-experts -missing-from-the-ebola-response-anthropologists

Kenyon, J. (2017, January 29). At the Shady Lawn Motel, every room has a story. *Valley News.* https://www.vnews.com/More-to-Shady-Lawn-Motel-Than-Meets-the -Eye-7727873

Keys to the Valley. (2022). 2010 housing needs forecast. Retrieved May 7, 2022, from https://www.keystothevalley.com/report/2030-home-projections/#:~:text=It%20 is%20estimated%20that%20approximately,in%20the%20number%20of%20 households

Kleinman, A. (1980). *Patients and healers in the context of culture: An exploration of the borderland between anthropology, medicine, and psychiatry* (Vol. 3). University of California Press.

Kleinman, A. (1988). *The illness narratives: Suffering, healing and the human condition.* Basic Books.

Kleinman, A. (1995). *Writing at the margin: Discourse between anthropology and medicine.* University of California Press.

Kleinman, A. (1998). Experience and its moral modes: Culture, human conditions, and disorder. Tanner Lectures on Human Values, Stanford University.

Kleinman, A. (2007). *What really matters: Living a moral life amidst uncertainty and danger.* Oxford University Press.

Kozol, J. (2011). *Rachel and her children: Homeless families in America.* Crown.

Lam, J. A., & Rosenheck, R. (1999). Street outreach for homeless persons with serious mental illness: Is it effective? *Medical Care, 37*(9), 894–907.

Lambek, M. (Ed.). (2010). *Ordinary ethics: Anthropology, language, and action.* Fordham University Press.

Lawrence, M. (1995). Rural homelessness: A geography without geography. *Journal of Rural Studies, 11*(3), 297–307.

LeVine, R. (1982). *Culture, behavior, and personality: An introduction to the comparative study of psycho-social adaptation* (2nd ed.). Aldine.

Levy, R. I., & Hollan, D. W. (2015). Person-centered interviewing and observation. In H. R. Bernard & C. C. Gravlee (Eds.), *Handbook of methods in cultural anthropology* (pp. 313–342). Rowman and Littlefield.

Lindsey, E. W. (1996). Mothers' perceptions of factors influencing the restabilization of homeless families. *Families in Society, 77*(4), 203–215.

Lipsky, M. (2010). *Street-level bureaucracy: Dilemmas of the individual in public service.* Russell Sage Foundation. (Original work published in 1980)

Liu, M., Luong, L., Lachaud, J., Edalati, H., Reeves, A., & Hwang, S. W. (2021). Adverse childhood experiences and related outcomes among adults experiencing homelessness: A systematic review and meta-analysis. *The Lancet Public Health, 6*(11), e836–e847.

Lo, E., Balasuriya, L., & Steiner, J. L. (2021). A street psychiatry rotation for medical trainees: Humanizing the care of people experiencing homelessness. *Academic Psychiatry, 46*(2), 1–6.

Luhrmann, T. (2007). Social defeat and the culture of chronicity: Or, why schizophrenia does so well over there and so badly here. *Culture, Medicine and Psychiatry, 31*(2), 135–172.

Luhrmann, T. M. (2008). "The street will drive you crazy": Why homeless psychotic women in the institutional circuit in the United States often say no to offers of help. *American Journal of Psychiatry, 165*(1), 15–20.

Malik, R., Hamm, K., Schochet, L., Novoa, C., Workman, S., & Jessen-Howard, S. (2018). America's child care deserts in 2018. https://americanprogress.org/wp-content/uploads/2018/12/AmericasChildCareDeserts20182.pdf?_ga=2.61786412.1606237730.1655157979-700565307.1655157979

Markus, H. R., & Conner, A. (2013). *Clash! 8 cultural conflicts that make us who we are.* Hudson Street Press.

Marrow, J., & Luhrmann, T. M. (2012). The zone of social abandonment in cultural geography: On the street in the United States, inside the family in India. *Culture, Medicine and Psychiatry, 36*, 493–513.

Marti, J. E. (2016). *Starting fieldwork: Methods and experiences.* Waveland Press.

Mattingly, C. (1994). The concept of therapeutic "emplotment." *Social Science & Medicine, 38*(6), 811–822.

Mattingly, C. (2010). *The paradox of hope: Journey through a clinical borderland.* University of California Press.

Mattingly, C. (2014). *Moral laboratories: Family peril and the struggle for a good life.* University of California Press.

Mattingly, C. (2018). Ordinary possibility, transcendent immanence, and responsive ethics: A philosophical anthropology of the small event. *HAU: Journal of Ethnographic Theory, 8*(1–2), 172–184.

McQuistion, H. L., Ranz, J. M., & Gillig, P. M. (2004). A survey of American psychiatric residency programs concerning education in homelessness. *Academic Psychiatry, 28*(2), 116–121.

Meert, H., & Bourgeois, M. 2005. Between rural and urban slums: A geography of pathways through homelessness. *Housing Studies, 20*(1), 107–125.

Metzl, J. M., & Hansen, H. 2014. Structural competency: Theorizing a new medical engagement with stigma and inequality. *Social Science & Medicine, 103*, 126–133.

Mezzina, R., Davidson, L., Borg, M., Marin, I., Topor, A., & Sells, D. (2006). The social nature of recovery: Discussion and implications for practice. *American Journal of Psychiatric Rehabilitation, 9*, 63–80.

Miller, M. (2020, January 9). What you need to know about how Section 8 really works. *ProPublica.* https://www.propublica.org/article/what-you-need-to-know-about-how-section-8-really-works#what-to-know-about-the-voucher

Mishler, E. G. (1981). Viewpoint: Critical perspectives on the biomedical model. In E. G. Mishler, L. R. AmaraSingham, S. T. Hauser, R. Liem, S. D. Osherson, & N. E. Waxler (Eds.), *Social contexts of health, illness, and patient care* (pp. 1–23). Cambridge University Press.

Mor Barak, M. E., Nissly, J. A., & Levin, A. (2001). Antecedents to retention and turn-over among child welfare, social work, and other human service employees: What can we learn from past research? A review and metanalysis. *Social Service Review*, *75*(4), 625–661.

Moses, J. (2019). *Demographic data project. Part IV. The role of geography*. Homelessness Research Institute, National Alliance to End Homelessness. Retrieved June 28, 2021, from https://endhomelessness.org/wp-content/uploads/2019/09/DDP-Geography -brief-09272019-byline-single-pages.pdf

Mowbray, C., Oyserman, D., & Ross, S. (1995). Parenting and the significance of children for women with a serious mental illness. *Journal of Mental Health Adminis-tration*, *22*, 189–200.

Mowbray, C., Oyserman, D., Zemencuk, J. K., & Ross, S. R. (1995). Motherhood for women with serious mental illness: Pregnancy, childbirth, and the postpartum period. *American Journal of Orthopsychiatry*, *65*(1), 21–38.

Myers, N. L. (2015). *Recovery's edge: An ethnography of mental health care and moral agency*. Vanderbilt University Press.

Myers, N. L. (2016). Recovery stories: An anthropological exploration of moral agency in stories of mental health recovery. *Transcultural Psychiatry*, *53*(4), 427–444.

National Council on Disability. (2012). *Rocking the cradle: Ensuring the rights of parents with disabilities and their children*. https://ncd.gov/publications/2012/Sep272012/Ch5

National Low Income Housing Coalition. (2020). *Out of reach 2020: Vermont report*. https://reports.nlihc.org/oor/vermont

New Hampshire Bureau of Family Assistance. (2021, July). NH Bureau of Family Assis-tance fact sheet. https://www.dhhs.nh.gov/dfa/documents/fam-asst-fact-sheet.pdf

New Hampshire Coalition to End Homelessness. (2018, December 19). The state of homelessness in New Hampshire report: An examination of homelessness, related economic and demographic factors, and changes at the state and county levels. Manchester, NH. Retrieved October 5, 2022, from: https://www.nhceh.org/wp -content/uploads/2018/12/2018-Report.pdf

New Hampshire Economic & Labor Market Information Bureau. (2013). *Lebanon, NH—Community profile*. New Hampshire Employment Security. http://www.nhes.nh .gov/elmi/products/cp/profiles-htm/lebanon.htm

Nicholson, J. (2014). Supporting mothers living with mental illnesses in recovery. In *Motherhood, mental illness and recovery* (pp. 3–17). Springer.

Nicholson, J., Biebel, K., Hinden, B., Henry, A., & Stier, L. (2001). *Critical issues for parents with mental illness and their families*. Report prepared for the Center for Mental Health Services, Substance Abuse and Mental Health Services Administration.

Nicholson, J., Sweeney, E., & Geller, J. (1998). Focus on women: Mothers with mental illness: I. The competing demands of parenting and living with mental illness. *Psychiatric Services, 49*(5), 635–642.

Nord, M., & Luloff, A. E. (1988). Homeless children and their families in New Hampshire: A rural perspective. *Social Service Review, 69,* 461–478.

Ochs, E., & Capps, L. (1996). Narrating the self. *Annual Review of Anthropology, 25*(1), 19–43.

Ortner, S. B. (1998). The hidden life of class. *Journal of Anthropological Research, 54,* 1–17.

Padgett, D. K. (2007). There's no place like (a) home: Ontological security among persons with serious mental illness in the United States. *Social Science & Medicine, 64*(9), 1925–1936.

Padgett, D. K. (2012). *Qualitative and mixed methods in public health.* Sage.

Parish, S. (2008). *Subjectivity and suffering in American culture: Possible selves.* Springer.

Park, J. M., Solomon, P., & Mandell, D. (2006). Involvement in the child welfare system among mothers with serious mental illnesses. *Psychiatric Services, 57*(4), 493–497.

Patton, L. (1988). *The rural homeless.* National Center for Health Services Research.

Peng, Y., Hahn, R. A., Finnie, R. K., Cobb, J., Williams, S. P., Fielding, J. E., . . . & Community Preventive Services Task Force. (2020). Permanent supportive housing with housing first to reduce homelessness and promote health among homeless populations with disability: A community guide systematic review. *Journal of Public Health Management and Practice, 26*(5), 404–411.

Poremski, D., Whitley, R., & Latimer, E. (2016). Building trust with people receiving supported employment and housing first services. *Psychiatric Rehabilitation Journal, 39*(1), 20.

Robbins, J. (2013). Beyond the suffering subject: Toward an anthropology of the good. *Journal of the Royal Anthropological Institute, 19*(3), 447–462.

Roberts, D. (2021). Abolish family policing, too. *Dissent, 68*(3), 67–69.

Roberts, D. (2022). *Torn apart: How the child welfare system destroys black families—and how abolition can build a safer world.* Basic Books.

Sermons, M. W., & Witte, P. (2011). *State of homelessness in America, January 2011.* National Alliance to End Homelessness.

Shamblin, S. R., Williams, N. F., & Bellaw, J. R. (2012). Conceptualizing homelessness in rural Appalachia: Understanding contextual factors relevant to community mental health practice. *Journal of Rural Mental Health, 36*(2), 3–9.

Shaw, M. (2004). Housing and public health. *Annual Review of Public Health, 25,* 397–418.

Sherman, J. (2006). Coping with rural poverty: Economic survival and moral capital in rural America. *Social Forces, 85*(2), 891–913.

Shohet, M., & Anderson, E. (2017). Virtuous families? Defining, enacting, or treating (im)moral families in everyday and institutional contexts. Session at the Biennial Meeting of the Society for Psychological Anthropology, New Orleans, March 10.

Smedley, B. D., Stith, A. Y., & Nelson, A. R. (Eds.), & Institute of Medicine, Committee on Understanding and Eliminating Racial and Ethnic Disparities in Health Care. (2003). *Unequal treatment: Confronting racial and ethnic disparities in healthcare.* National Academies Press.

Snell-Rood, C., & Carpenter-Song, E. (2018). Depression in a depressed area: Deservingness, mental illness, and treatment in the contemporary rural US. *Social Science & Medicine, 219*, 78–86.

Snow, D. A., Anderson, L., & Koegel, P. (1994). Distorting tendencies in research on the homeless. *American Behavioral Scientist, 37*(4), 461–475.

Sosin, A., & Carpenter-Song, E. (2020). Village vs. virus: Rural ethos protects where public health fails. *Health Affairs Blog*, July 27. DOI: 10.1377/hblog20200722.490817

Sosin, A., Carpenter-Song, E., Griffin, M., & O'Reilly, M. (2021). Housing is health: Building on Vermont's pandemic success to advance health equity. Legislative Brief submitted to the Vermont General Assembly, January 24.

Spradley, J. P. (2016). *Participant observation.* Waveland Press. (Original work published in 1980)

Stack, C. (1974). *All our kin: Strategies for survival in a Black community.* Basic Books.

State of Vermont Judiciary. (2017). *Vermont judiciary annual statistical report FY 2016.* https://www.vermontjudiciary.org/sites/default/files/documents/FY16%20Statisti cal%20Report%20-%20FINAL%20020617_1.pdf

Stein, L. I., & Santos, A. B. (1998). *Assertive community treatment of persons with severe mental illness.* Norton.

Stefancic, A., Henwood, B. F., Melton, H., Shin, S. M., Lawrence-Gomez, R., & Tsemberis, S. (2013). Implementing housing first in rural areas: Pathways Vermont. *American Journal of Public Health, 103*(S2), S206–S209.

Strauss, C. (2000). The culture concept and the individualism-collectivism debate: Dominant and alternative attributions for class in the United States. In L. P. Nucci, G. B. Saxe, & E. Turiel (Eds.), *Culture, thought, and development* (pp. 85–114). Lawrence Erlbaum Associates.

Substance Abuse and Mental Health Services Administration (SAMHSA). (2004). *National consensus statement on mental health recovery.* U.S. Department of Health and Human Services.

Thomas, K. C., Ellis, A. R., Konrad, T. R., Holzer, C. E., & Morrissey, J. P. (2009). County-level estimates of mental health professional shortage in the United States. *Psychiatric Services, 60*(10), 1323–1328. PMID: 19797371

Thomas, D., MacDowell, M., & Glasser, M. (2012). Rural mental health workforce needs assessment: A national survey. *Rural Remote Health, 12*(4), 1–12. PMID: 23088609

Tischler, V., Rademeyer, A., & Vostanis, P. 2007. Mothers experiencing homelessness: Mental health, support and social care needs. *Health and Social Care in the Community, 15,* 246–253.

Tree, C. (2014, August 4). The "Upper Valley": A place of unexpected discoveries. *Yankee.* https://newengland.com/yankee-magazine/travel/new-england/vacations/upper-valley/

Tsemberis, S. (1999). From streets to homes: An innovative approach to supported housing for homeless adults with psychiatric disabilities. *Journal of Community Psychology, 27*(2), 225–241.

Tsemberis, S., & Eisenberg, R. F. (2000). Pathways to housing: Supported housing for street-dwelling homeless individuals with psychiatric disabilities. *Psychiatric Services, 51*(4), 487–493.

Union Leader. (2011, March 30). NH homeless tops 2,500.

U.S. Census. (2019). Quickfacts: Hanover, New Hampshire. Population estimates July 1, 2019. Retrieved October 27, 2020, from https://www.census.gov/quickfacts/hanovercdpnewhampshire.

U.S. Census. (2020a). Quickfacts: Hartford, Vermont. Population estimates April 1, 2020. Retrieved October 27, 2020, from https://www.census.gov/quickfacts/fact/table/hartfordtownwindsorcountyvermont/PST040219

U.S. Census. (2020b). Quickfacts: New Hampshire, Vermont. Retrieved June 29, 2021, from https://www.census.gov/quickfacts/fact/table/NH,VT,US/PST045219.

U.S. Department of Health and Human Services. (2001). *Mental health: Culture, race, ethnicity.* Supplement to *Mental health: Report of the surgeon general.* Rockville, MD.

U.S. Department of Housing and Urban Development (HUD). (2021). CoC homeless populations and subpopulations reports. HUD Exchange. https://www.hudexchange.info/programs/coc/coc-homeless-populations-and-subpopulations-reports/?filter_Year=2020&filter_Scope=&filter_State=&filter_CoC=&program=CoC&group=PopSub

Vermont Coalition to End Homelessness. (2020). *2020 Point-in-Time report: Everyone counts, no matter where they live.* Retrieved October 12, 2022, from https://helpingtohousevt.org/wp-content/uploads/2020/06/2020-PIT-Report-FINAL-1.pdf

Vermont Housing Finance Agency. (2012). *Annual report.* Burlington, VT. http://www.leg.state.vt.us/reports/2013ExternalReports/286439.pdf

Vermont Housing Finance Agency. (2018). *Renter cost burden*. Retrieved October 28, 2020, from https://www.housingdata.org/profile/rental-housing-costs/renter-cost -burden

Vermont State Government. (2013). *Towns and counties–Vershire*. Retrieved September 23, 2013, from http://vermont.gov/portal/government/towns.php?town=215

Vissing, Y. M. (1996). *Out of sight, out of mind: Homeless children and families in small-town America*. University Press of Kentucky.

Wagner, J. D., Menke, E. M., & Ciccone, J. K. (1995). What is known about the health of rural homeless families? *Public Health Nursing, 12*(6), 400–408.

Walsh, Molly. (2016, May 11). Why more Vermont parents are losing their children—Permanently. *Seven Days*. https://www.sevendaysvt.com/vermont/why-more-vermont -parents-are-losing-their-children-permanently/Content?oid=3349530

Wallner, M. J. (2017, June 5). Children in need caught in a perfect storm. *New Hampshire Business Review*. http://nhbr.com/children-in-need-caught-in-a-perfect-storm

Wang, P. S., Lane, M., Olfson, M., Pincus, H. A., Wells, K.B., & Kessler, R. C. 2005. Twelve-month use of mental health services in the United States: Results from the national comorbidity survey replication. *Archives of General Psychiatry, 62*(6), 629–640.

Watkins, M. (2015). Psychosocial accompaniment. *Journal of Social and Political Psychology, 3*(1), 324–341.

White House. (n.d.). The child tax credit. Retrieved October 12, 2022, from https://www .whitehouse.gov/child-tax-credit/#:~:text=has%20for%20you.-,How%20much%20 will%20I%20receive%20in%20Child%20Tax%20Credit%20payments,child%20 ages%206%20to%2017

Whitley, R. (2013). Fear and loathing in New England: Examining the health-care perspectives of homeless people in rural areas. *Anthropology & Medicine, 20*(3), 232–243.

Whitley, R. (2014). Beyond critique: Rethinking roles for the anthropology of mental health. *Culture, Medicine and Psychiatry, 38*(3), 499–511.

Willen, S. S. (2012). How is health-related "deservingness" reckoned? Perspectives from unauthorized im/migrants in Tel Aviv. *Social Science & Medicine, 74*(6), 812–821.

Williams, Raymond. (1989). *The resources of hope: Culture, democracy, socialism*. London: Verso.

Zigon, J. (2014). Attunement and fidelity: Two ontological conditions for morally being-in-the world. *Ethos, 42*(1), 16–30.

Zigon, J., & Throop, J. (2014). Moral experience: Introduction. *Ethos, 42*(1), 1–15.

Zimmer, B. (2005). Figurative "bootstraps." Listserv posting. Retrieved August 29, 2021, http://listserv.linguistlist.org/pipermail/ads-l/2005-August/052756.html

Index